CBD & HEMP OIL ALCHEMY

HEALING THROUGH CBD OIL & HEMP MANAGING SEVERE PAIN TO DEPRESSION

HOW TO EXTRACT CBD AND HEMP OIL, WHAT ILLNESSES THEY CAN ACTUALLY HEAL, WHAT THE PROPER DOSAGES ARE, HOW TO USE EACH OIL, RECIPES OF GOURMET DESSERTS TO SKIN CARE PRODUCTS YOU CAN MAKE WITH EACH OIL.

By

Robert R. Sanders

Published by:

Lost River Publishing House

Cover & Interior designed

By

Jason Roberts

First Edition

<u>**Legal Disclaimer**</u>

This book contains information about controlled and illegal substances, especially the plant Cannabis and its derivative products. River of Lakes Publishing Press emphasizes that Cannabis and its derivative products are considered controlled substance in the US and throughout most of the world. As such, use of such products where it is against the law is not implied or suggested.

The aim of the publisher is to educate and to entertain only. The readers should use and enjoy suggested ways of enjoying Cannabis only where it is legal by the law.

Inside This Book

WHAT IS CBD AND HEMP OIL

The cannabis oil industry is very dynamic and fast-growing. It created a new category of products made with CBD hemp oil that is becoming widely popular. CBD oil is made from hemp that is made from high-CBD and low-THC hemp. It is that fact that makes it very different from medical marijuana products. Those products are made from the types of plants that have high concentrations of psychoactive tetrahydrocannabinol, or THC.

The abbreviation CBD is fully pronounced cannabidiol. It is just one of the 85 cannabinoids that can be identified in the cannabis plant, but it is only second to THC in its prominence in marijuana. It has a minimal amount of THC and a considerable amount of CBD. CBD is found in the flowers, leaves, and stalks of the Cannabis plant.

CBD is a substance that does not give you any high or euphoric feeling. This is because of the low amount of THC. It is also found growing in all parts of the world and is imported into the US, where it is used in many nutritional products and foods. CBD is used to treat a variety of illnesses, conditions, and their symptoms. Choosing CBD oil over other methods of pain relief, or as a complement to them, is a great option for anyone. This book's goal is to provide you with high-quality information to make informed decisions.

Hemp oil is extracted from the hemp plant. Plants in the Cannabis genus can produce oil. Hemp oil is typically very close to being free of THC, and it has no psychoactive properties.

They tend to produce the very best hemp oil, but the whole plant can be pressed to extract the oil. The hemp oil you make at home will be unrefined. Unrefined hemp oil does not have a very long shelf life. The oil quickly goes bad. The only way to preserve it is to store it in dark containers in a refrigerated environment. People who use unrefined hemp oil generally purchase it in small amounts so that it will not go bad.

Both CBD and Hemp are very controversial in some regions of the world; this is because of concerns about psychoactive plants in the Cannabis genus. In some regions, cultivation of hemp is banned, although products made from hemp, such as the oil or hemp paper, may be legal.

In other areas, hemp is legal, but only industrial hemp, so home growing or extraction is illegal in most states. Then there are others that freely permit the cultivation of all of these types of plants.

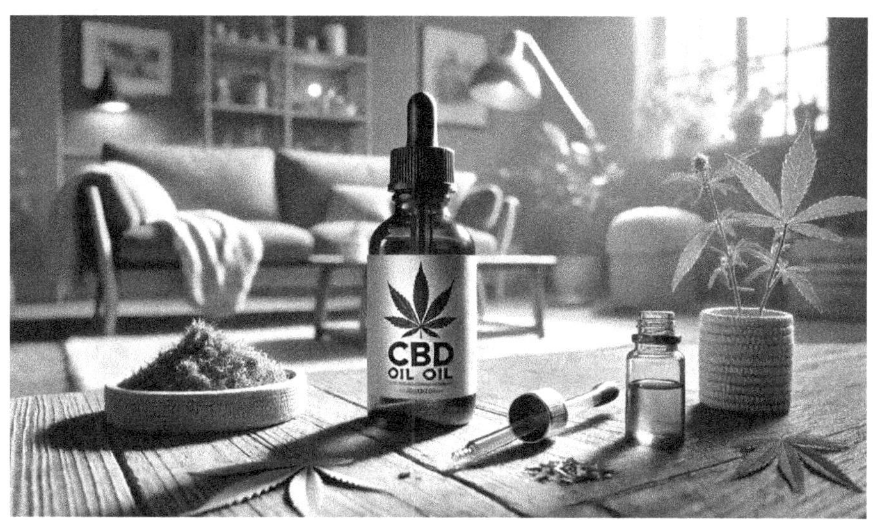

CBD
OIL OIL

Origins of CBD

So far, science has identified 86 cannabinoids in both the natural marijuana plant and chemically synthesized cannabinoids. The main psychoactive ingredient in marijuana is the delta-9-tetrahydrocannabinol, referred to as THC (this is the part that gives people the "high" feeling).

Other cannabinoids have medicinal, psychoactive, or both effects. Some of these include Cannabidiol (CBD), Cannabinol (CBN), Cannabavarin (THCV), Cannabigerol (CBG), Cannabichromene (CBC), THC, Cannabicyclol (CBL), Cannabitriol (CBT) and Cannabielsoin; among others.

THC

Since THC is the main psychoactive compound in marijuana, it is often used to measure the herb's potency. The typical concentrations for THC are as follows:

➢ Inactive hemp - Less than 0.5%

➢ Marijuana leaf - 2 to 3%

➢ Higher-grade marijuana - 4 to 20%

The highest concentrations of THC are found in seedless buds known as sinsemilla. You can also get high concentrations of THC in extracts, tonics, and hashish or concentrated cannabis resin.

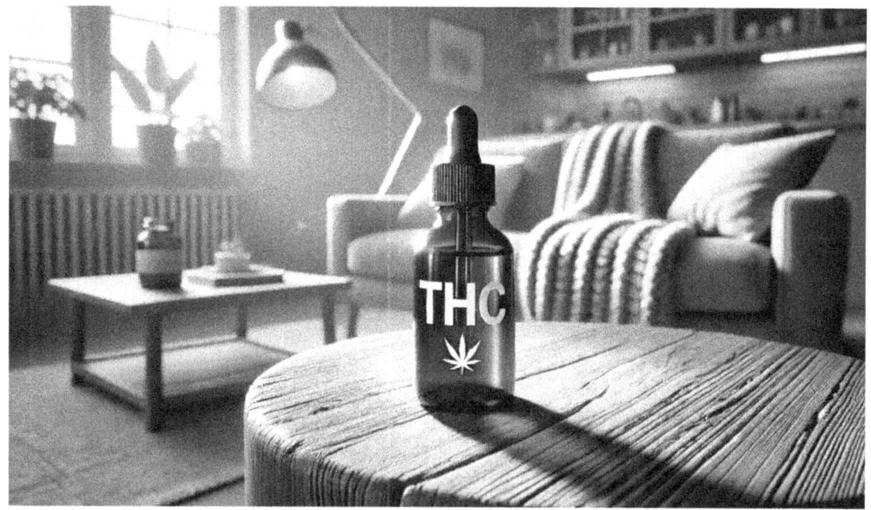

THC doesn't naturally occur in its active form within the cannabis plant. Instead, it happens in an acidic form known as tetrahydrocannabinolic acid or THC acid (THCA). The THCA is converted to THC when burned in a cigarette or heated in cooking through a heat-propelled reaction called decarboxylation.

Eating raw marijuana won't have any substantial psychoactive effects because the THCA is inactive.

However, as the plant ages, some THCA undergoes decarboxylation.

I know it sounded boring for me to mention all those long-winded names, but stay with me, and it will get more interesting, I promise.

CBD

This is the second most common cannabinoid and is the most prevalent in hemp varieties of cannabis. CBD lacks any noticeable psychoactive effects and doesn't interact with the body's cannabinoid receptors. However, there is ample evidence that CBD has medicinal properties.

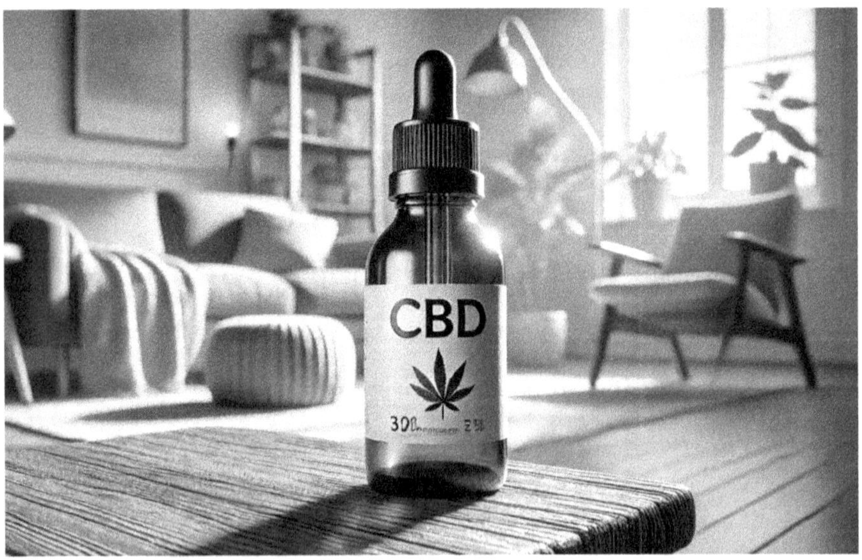

CBD will also work along with THC to augment its medicinal effects while moderating the psychoactive effects. Researchers have also found that CBD has antipsychotic properties, which reduce anxiety and panic reactions associated with THC.

Although CBD can be taken by itself for some medicinal benefits that I'll discuss later. However, the evidence does show that CBD is biphasic, meaning the effectiveness can be diminished if the dose is either too low or too high.

CBD and THC acid are simultaneously produced. In the marijuana plant, the precursor for both is a cannabinoid called Cannabigerolic acid. Each cannabinoid is produced by a different enzyme that acts on the Cannabigerolic acid.

This means it is hard to find a plant that has a high level of both CBD and THC. Depending on the breed type, some marijuana plants are naturally high on THC while relatively low on CBD and vice versa. Generally, as you can imagine, people always seek the type that is high in THC, as that is what gives them the desired "high".

Lately, some of the hydroponic marijuana strains are gaining popularity for their highly potent THC level.

Hemp plants will often lack the enzyme that produces THC, so CBD is often prevalent. However, most consumer-grade marijuana has significantly low levels of CBD since growers selectively breed out the CBD enzyme in favor of producing more THC-potent breeds (since that is what people want, and that is where the money is).

CBN

The third most common (out of 80 or so) cannabinoid found in marijuana is CBN. This is a byproduct of the chemical breakdown of THC.

CBN lacks both the strong medicinal and psychoactive qualities of THC and is often only found in degraded or poorly-preserved marijuana plants.

As you may have heard, cannabis is widely used as a sleep aid. CBN (cannabinol) is the part of cannabis that is responsible for the sedative effects. This is also why CBN is the third most popular cannabinoid out of so many of its components.

CBD Oil for Pain Management

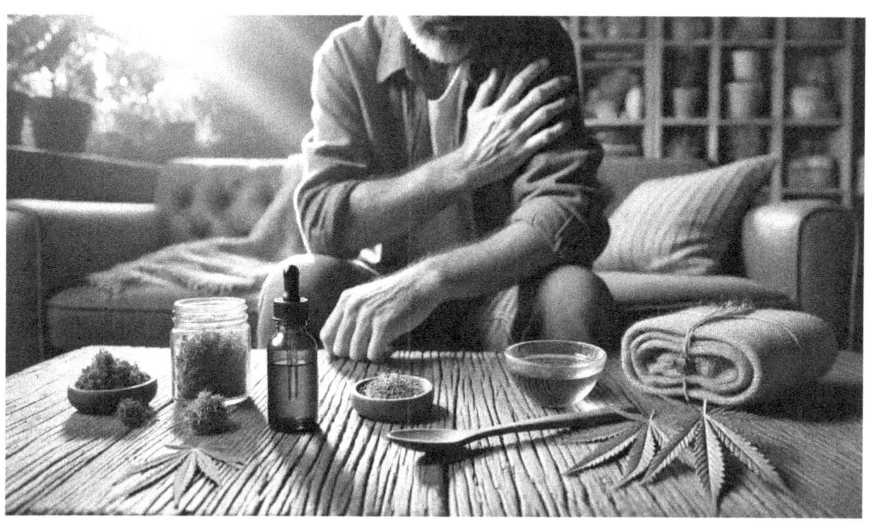

Pain management, both acute and chronic, can be hard to manage and/or treat. As the population starts to age, millions are starting to suffer from chronic pain. Causes of pain can range from arthritis to side effects of cancer. Consider some facts related to pain:

- One-fifth of adults over 65 experience pain that lasts over 24 hours.
- Three-fifths of adults over 65 experience pain that lasts a year or more.
- One-quarter of adults suffer from low back pain.

- 15% of adults experience severe or migraine headaches.

Commonly, people turn to opioids to help with chronic pain. Not only do these medications come with a risk of addiction, but they can also have side effects such as constipation, nausea, and ulcers. This is why cannabinoids are becoming popular.

It is so effective that some doctors are even prescribing it instead of traditional pain medications. Not to mention, this is the best natural pain reliever with no harsh side effects.

CBD VS. THC: WHICH STOPS PAIN BEST?

When it comes to CBD and THC, they both stop the pain. Each compound has pain-fighting properties, and they actually work best when consumed together. Both CBD and THC work together to enhance the pain-fighting effects of the herb. However, THC is the main psychoactive component of the cannabis plant and consuming this compound isn't for everyone. You'll likely need to do some experimenting to determine the type of cannabis that works best for your unique pain situation.

CBD is not psychoactive like THC, but it still has similar effects on the brain. However, CBD won't cause the same noticeable "high" feeling as THC. Rather, CBD is a cannabinoid that has calming and uplifting effects, helping reduce pain and inflammation. Often, high CBD strains work best for the pain that comes from spasticity and cramping. Research often shows that the best pain management comes from strains with high amounts of both compounds.

WHY CBD OIL VS. PAINKILLERS

Prescription painkillers and other drugs present some dangers. Prescription painkillers can become addictive and lead to some symptoms, including the following:

- Irritability
- Sleep disruption
- Digestive complications
- Increase risk of suicide

CBD oil has become popular because it doesn't come with these serious side effects. Before you can start considering using CBD oil for pain relief, you first need to understand what CBD oil is and how it works in your body.

The best way to know what CBD oil is to know where it comes from. CBD is a cannabinoid-like THC that comes from the cannabis (marijuana) plant. CBD or cannabidiol is a natural chemical found within the cannabis plant.

CBD is a substance that is non-psychoactive, unlike THC. CBD provides relaxation without any intoxicating effects. CBD is the second most prominent compound found in the cannabis plant. Many of the health benefits associated with THC are a result of the CBD content.

How CBD Develops

The starting material is Cannabigerolic acid (CBGa). This leads to strains of CBDa, THCa, and CBCa. When CBGa is present in sufficient amounts, it will convert to CBDa. This is CBD with a carboxylic acid group attached. Through heat or time, the carboxylic acid is naturally released from the compound, converting it into CBD. This process happens at about 80 degrees Celsius.

What Are Cannabinoids?

Cannabinoids are one of the most important groups of active compounds within the cannabis plant. The plant itself has over 500 compounds; cannabinoids make up about 85 of them. The other compounds consist of terpenes, vitamins, minerals, proteins, and chlorophyll.

HOW DOES IT WORK?

The endocannabinoid system communicates directly with receptors in the body and brain, altering the way pain is perceived. The human body naturally produces chemical cannabinoids to regulate body functions. This is likely why CBD provides good results. Let's look at how CBD works within the body.

Healing with CBD Oil

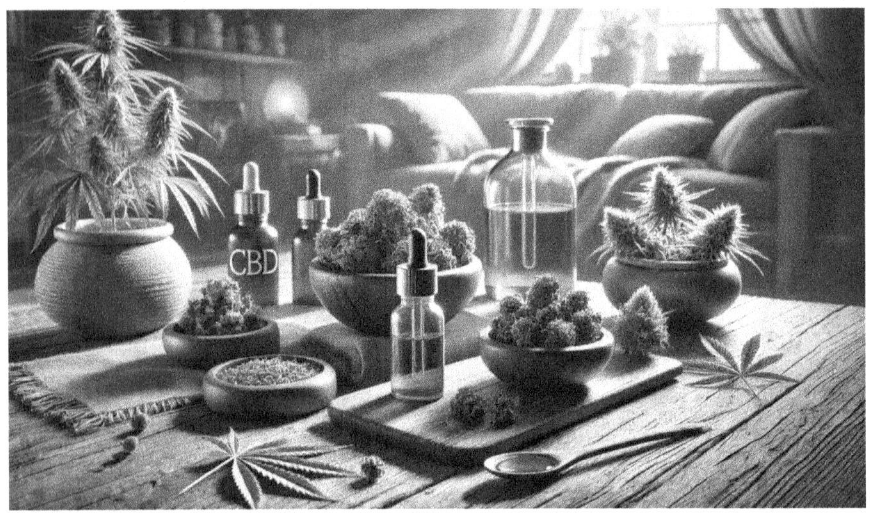

CBD, or cannabidiol, is one of 60 compounds known as cannabinoids. Cannabinoids are found in a number of plants, but are commonly associated with cannabis. Unlike other popular cannabinoids such as THC (tetrahydrocannabinol), CBD doesn't produce the "high" or psychoactive effect. This is because CBD doesn't affect the same receptors that THC does.

The endocannabinoid system in the human body receives and translates signals from cannabinoids. The body produces some cannabinoids on its own, known as endocannabinoids. The endocannabinoid system helps regulate functions such as sleep, immune system responses, and pain.

THC gives an individual a "high" feeling as it interacts with the brain's endocannabinoid receptors. This triggers the brain's reward system and produces pleasure-related chemicals, such as dopamine. CBD is a distinct compound with complex effects on the body.

It isn't psychoactive, so it doesn't produce the "high" feeling or change a person's state of mind. Rather, it influences the body to use its own endocannabinoids more effectively. A study found that this is because CBD does little to the endocannabinoid system beyond activating or inhibiting other compounds within the system.

For example, CBD prevents the body from absorbing anandamide, a compound often associated with pain regulation. Having increased levels of anandamide in the blood can reduce how much pain a person feels.

Cannabidiol can also limit inflammation within the brain and nervous system, helping those who experience pain, insomnia, and other immune-system responses.

Now that we know how CBD works in the body, just what can it do for you? CBD can help with the following conditions and more:

* Alzheimer's
* Anorexia
* Anxiety
* Arthritis
* Asthma
* Bipolar Disorder
* Cancer
* Cardiovascular Conditions
* Chronic Pain
* Depression
* Epilepsy
* Glaucoma
* Huntington's Disease
* Inflammation
* Insomnia
* Multiple Sclerosis
* Nausea
* Obesity
* Parkinson's Disease
* PTSD

* ★ Schizophrenia

* ★ Tourette's Syndrome

Consider all the benefits that CBD offers and you'll see why it works for such an extensive list of conditions.

TYPES OF PAIN MANAGED BY CBD OIL

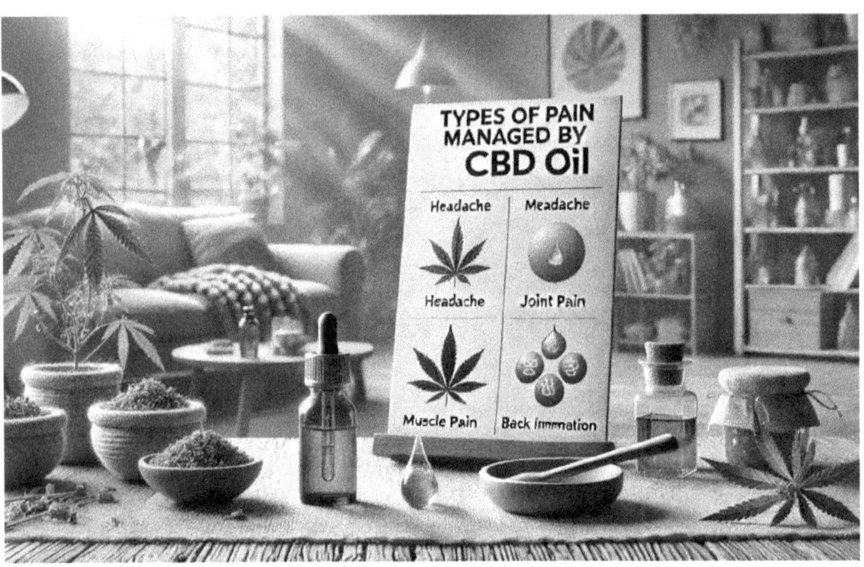

For thousands of years, CBD oil has been a traditional treatment for many types of pain. However, it hasn't been until recently that scientists have begun studying it again. Consider some recent research into the benefits of CBD oil.

ARTHRITIS PAIN

The European Journal of Pain published an animal study examining whether CBD oil could help with arthritis pain. A topical gel of CBD was applied to rats with arthritis for four days. The results showed a significant reduction in signs of inflammation and pain, without any additional side effects. While these results are promising, there have been no human studies to confirm them yet.

MULTIPLE SCLEROSIS

MS, or Multiple Sclerosis, is an autoimmune disorder that affects the entire body, particularly the brain and nerves. One of the most common symptoms of MS is muscle spasms. For some people, these spasms are so great that they can cause constant pain. A study found that short-term use of CBD oil can reduce the level of spasticity in people. While the results were modest, many people reported a reduction in symptoms. These results need to be verified with additional human studies.

CHRONIC PAIN

The same report as that for MS also studied CBD for use in general chronic pain. Researchers compiled results from several systematic reviews that covered a range of trials and studies. The research found that there was ample evidence to prove that cannabis is an effective treatment for chronic pain in adults.

The Journal of Experimental Medicine did a separate study that supports these results. Research suggests that CBD use can reduce pain and inflammation. The research also found that people were not likely to build up a tolerance to the effects of CBD, so that they wouldn't require an increase in dosage over time. The researchers noted that cannabinoids like CBD could be a helpful new treatment for those with chronic pain.

Apart from its effectiveness, CBD oil is also very easy to take. CBD oil can also treat a number of painful conditions rather than simply masking the pain.

MEDICAL RESEARCH

Several studies have shown that CBD oil can treat a range of medical conditions. The most well-known studies are those of CBD's effect on cancer and seizures. However, other studies have been just as promising.

A study in 2011 focused on CBD in fibromyalgia patients. The results: 56 of 112 participants experienced a significant reduction in pain and symptoms, while those on traditional treatments showed little improvement.

In addition to these benefits, there are very few side effects associated with CBD oil. I will talk about some of those in a later chapter.

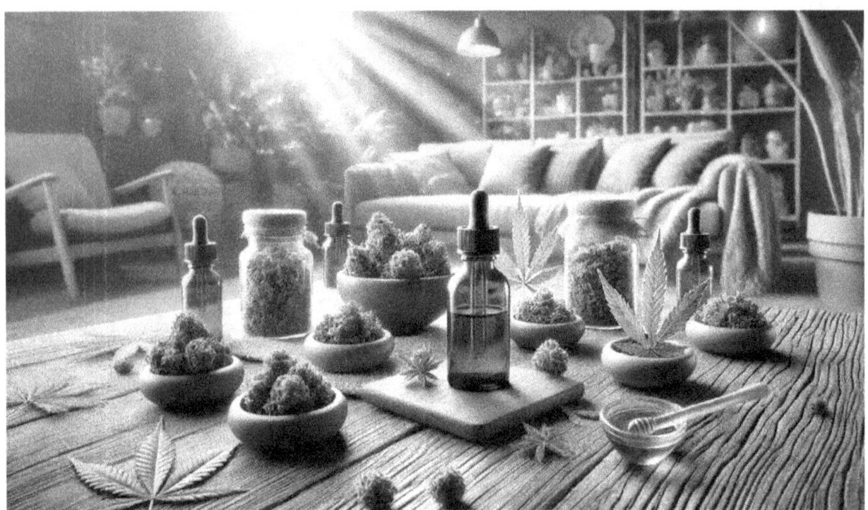

CBD is a cannabinoid found in the cannabis plant that has incredible potential to become a powerful alternative medicine for a wide range of illnesses. While CBD doesn't create psychoactive effects like other compounds found within the cannabis plant, the scientific and medical community still wants to do additional research to find out about the benefits of CBD and its effects on overall human health.

However, even without advanced research and studies, those who have tried CBD products for a range of pain and other health conditions, such as stress, anxiety, chronic pain, epilepsy and others, have claimed to have spectacular effects.

Add to this the fact that CBD has no risks associated with its use and consumption, you have a true natural product made from entirely extracted plant material. While the fact remains that there are some people who choose to use cannabis because of the "high" feeling, it is important to know that there are strains with high contents of CBD that give you therapeutic benefits without any "high" feeling.

While there are strains of the cannabis plant cultivated for their high THC content to provide the psychoactive effects some look for in recreational use, the following strains we are going to discuss are those that are high in CBD, so they are good options when you want to make your own CBD oil at home.

VARIOUS CANNABIS STRAINS WITH HIGH CBD CONCENTRATION

There are many excellent cannabis plants to choose from when considering extracting your own CBD, but there are several strains that are best for extraction. In today's market, there are many great choices. This section will lay out some great options and walk you through the benefits of each.

1. HARLEQUIN

This high-CBD strain is a great option to extract CBD from. It has an earthy smell with a hint of oak. It also has a subtle fruity sweetness. Harlequin is a Sativa-dominant strain. It works to ease anxiety and increase your alertness. It has a blend of cannabinoids that really complement each other, making it an excellent option for pain management. It is very commonly used for migraine sufferers due to its quick-acting pain relief. It has a CBD/THC ratio of 5:2.

2. RINGO'S GIFT

This strain is actually a hybrid of the Harle-Tsu and AC-DC strains. This mixture makes it almost completely THC-free. The ratio is 24:1 CBD/THC. It has a piney, citrusy smell. Because it has such a high amount of CBD, the pain relief is extremely fast, faster than any other strain on this list. It can also really reduce inflammation. Inflammation is one of the causes of so many different ailments, such as headaches and muscle pain. The only problem with this strain is that it is less available than other strains

3. SWEET AND SOUR WIDOW

This strain is actually White Widow strain that has been enriched with CBD. It has a 1:1 CBD/THC ratio. It has a sweet-to-woodsy ratio. It can work to reduce pain. This strain works great for insomnia, helping you relax and sleep, thereby relieving fatigue. Those with depression also tend to turn to this strain for the relief of their symptoms.

4. STEPHEN HAWKING KUSH

This strain is an Indica-dominant hybrid. It has a fruity and minty smell. It works great for those who regularly have stomach aches because it stimulates your stomach to suppress nausea. It has a 5:1 CBD-to-THC ratio. It also can reduce stress while helping you relax without making you sleepy. That makes this the perfect daytime strain to use for CBD oil.

5. AC/DC

This strain is also Sativa-dominant. It is a CBD/THC ratio of this strain that has been known to treat the very severe symptoms of multiple sclerosis and epilepsy. Medicines used to treat those symptoms can have harsh side effects.

CBD oil can really help without having to deal with prescriptions and risking feeling worse due to side effects.

6. CATATONIC

This unique hybrid is a mixture of MK Ultra and G13 Haze. It's particularly great for those who suffer from anxiety. Using this strain will lead you to feel a significantly higher level of relaxation. Its name can sound a bit scary, but its effect is happy, uplifting feelings. These feelings will naturally reduce the stress or fatigue you might be feeling. It can also help those seeking a boost of energy during the day.

7. HARLE-TSU

This strain is a hybrid of Harlequin and Sour Tsunami, with a CBD/THC ratio of 20:1. It has a citrus and woody aroma. Those with chronic depression have responded well when using CBD oil from this strain. It promotes relaxation and can even help you sleep during times when it's difficult.

8. SOUR TSUNAMI

This strain is actually one of the first strains grown specifically for CBD rather than THC. Those with high amounts of stress or depression would really benefit from this train. It works in your body to bring forth feelings of relaxation that can leave you with a positive outlook. Its smell is very sweet, which will appeal to more people than other strains.

9. PENNYWISE

This strain is for those with insomnia symptoms and chronic pain. It is a mixture of Harlequin and Jack the Ripper. It has a peppery smell. It has a higher amount of THC than some of the other strains. The CBD/THC ratio is 1:1.

Here's a handy chart of the best strains for CBD oil.

Cannabis Strain	Best Benefit	Fragrance
Harlequin	Decreases Pain and anxiety	Earthy, Sweet, and Woody
Ringo's Gift	Reduces pain and Inflammation	Earthy, Citrus, and Pine

Sweet and Sour Window	Reduces Insomnia symptoms and Fatigue	Earthy, Sweet, and Woody
Stephen Hawking Kush	Increases Relaxation and Reduces Stress	Earthy, Woody, and Berry
ACDC	Reduces Inflammation and Stress	Earthy, Woody, and Pine
Catatonic	Reduces Stress and General Pain	Earthy, Sweet, and Pine
Harle-TSU	Increase Metal Focus and Relaxation	Earthy, Citrus, and Woody
Sour Tsunami	Increases Relaxation and Overall, Happiness	Citrus, Diesel, and Earthy
Pennywise	Reduces Insomnia Symptoms and pain	Earthy, Woody, and Sweet

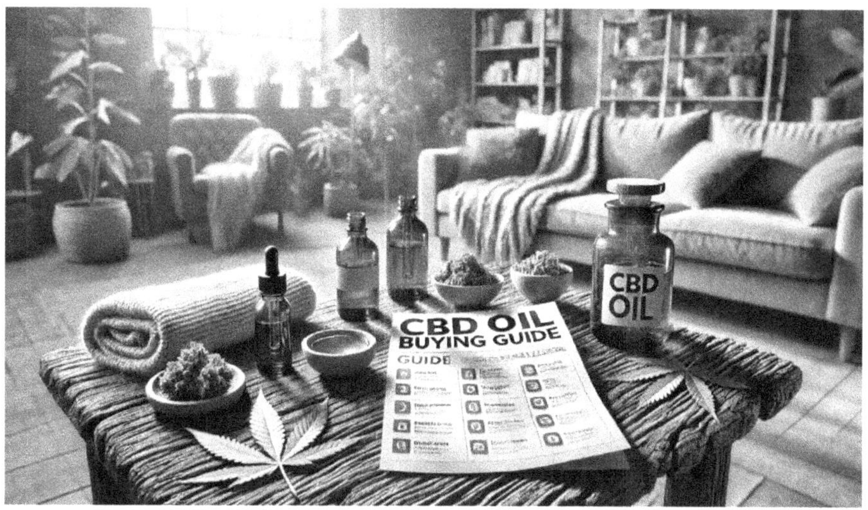

While you are likely to choose to make your own CBD oil since it is easy and saves you a great deal of money, some may still find it simpler to buy CBD oil. If you choose to purchase CBD oil, you will need to know a few things to buy the right one. Let's look at what you need to know and what you need to buy to get CBD oil.

CBD is easily one of the most misunderstood dietary supplements in today's healthcare market. A lot of it has to do with entrepreneurs coming into the market who try to sell the wrong cannabis strains. The other misunderstanding comes from the psychoactive legacy that is attached to the cannabis plant. Therefore, the first step is to make sure you know what to look for and who to shop from, something you are already doing by reading this guide.

If you are new to CBD oil and its related products, then you should keep reading this guide to help you in buying your first CBD oil product before you venture out to make your own CBD oil. With this guide, you won't have to dig too far to get the right information you need.

It is important to start your search with the right perspective on the cannabis plant and herb. It isn't a dangerous plant or herb used for evil purposes. Rather, cannabis has been used in the healing process for a variety of conditions for centuries, and it is just now being proven through studies to be highly effective for a range of conditions and diseases.

In fact, the combined benefits of the cannabis plant are nearly 1000 times more than the single bad, psychoactive trait of THC. However, it is this one bad trait that has endangered the entire reputation of the cannabis plant and herb.

It is important that you distinguish your cannabinoids. It is important to note that, as cannabinoids, both CBD and THC offer excellent healing properties. The main thing that separates the two is the fact that CBD has no psychoactive properties while THC does. In fact, CBD actually works to neutralize the psychoactive effects of THC.

Even THC offers a range of healing properties that can help with a wide range of conditions and diseases. However, because THC has psychoactive properties, it can be very difficult to get governments to legalize it. CBD doesn't have the same legal issues because it isn't considered a psychoactive substance.

The key is to educate people about the entire realm of cannabis and the difference between cannabinoids. In general, people still don't completely understand cannabis and cannabinoids, thinking that they are all the same when they aren't. The only way CBD and THC are similar is in the health benefits they offer.

In most states and countries, with a few exceptions, THC is only legally available as medical cannabis or medical THC when prescribed by a medical practitioner. CBD products, on the other hand, are completely legal throughout the world. CBD is also completely safe to use since it not only lacks the psychoactive component but also because there is nothing in it that can harm you.

Before you simply go out and buy a CBD product or a cannabis strain to make your own CBD product, there are a few things you need to consider. You particularly need to consider the product brand, the concentration, the type of product you want and specifically what you need the product for. It is always better to make an educated purchase, so keep reading.

WHAT TO CONSIDER WHEN BUYING CBD OIL

The first thing you want to establish is your buying criteria. Buying CBD oil is more than just browsing your options, clicking a choice and paying for it. To begin with, there are a number of products to choose from.

For example, are you going to need to purchase drops or a spray? You'll also need to look at how much CBD is in each specific product. Often CBD products come in a range of concentrations. There are three important criteria you need to look for when buying CBD products.

The first thing you need to know is that the content of CBD will differ between products. CBD doesn't harm you, but you need to know how much you need to consume in order to use your CBD product. Also, most CBD products are measured by how much CBD oil they contain and by the specific type of CBD oil.

Therefore, when buying a CBD product, it is important to find out how much CBD it contains and check whether that amount is listed in mg or percent.

HEMP OIL CONTENT

In addition to measuring CBD content in CBD products, hemp oil content is also measured. The difference is that the CBD is often contained within the hemp oil. This means the CBD content will always be less than the hemp oil content. Hemp oil has its own benefits, but when you buy a product for the CBD content in it, then it makes sense to pay attention to how much CBD the product contains. You can use the following calculation to determine the CBD content of your product.

Let's say you have a bottle of CBD Hemp Oil that is 10 ml or 10 grams total of oil. The bottle indicates it has 6% CBD. The 10 grams equals 10,000 milligrams. 6% of 10,000 milligrams equals 600 milligrams of pure CBD in the product.

CONCENTRATION

The concentration is just as important as the content and goes hand in hand with the strength and quality of any CBD product.

While content refers to how much CBD is in an individual product, concentration refers to the strength of the CBD in the product. Products will vary in concentration, from normal to very high. The specific concentration you choose will depend on the product you plan to purchase and the amount of CBD you plan to take.

For first-time users, the recommended dosage is typically between 1 and 2 milligrams a day to start, and it is adjusted until the desired effect is achieved. However, depending on your physical makeup, such as weight, metabolism and body type, you may choose to start with a dose of 3 milligrams and then adjust as needed.

You can also choose to gradually increase your dose as your body gets more used to the CBD. Since CBD has no psychoactive or dangerous properties, you can safely increase the amount you take until you reach your ideal dosage.

The best dosing method is to start with two to three milligrams a day for a week, and then double the dose for another week, and continue in this fashion until you reach a point where you can feel that you are taking the proper amount of CBD for your unique condition.

TYPES OF CBD PRODUCTS

CBD in all forms is a constructive and healthy supplement to your diet and health regimen. It is extremely flexible, no matter what form you choose, and can be used in a variety of formats. The range of health benefits you can enjoy from CBD is well known to many people who have used the product.

You can find CBD in a variety of formats, from oil concentrates to edibles.

You can even get CBD in an easy to dose drops and tinctures, as well as other formats. You can even find a range of CBD-based pet products so your pets can be pain-free and enjoy the health benefits of CBD.

You can even find CBD oil in a variety of flavors, so you can find something to match any taste. Let's take a look at the various options you have available.

CBD OIL TINCTURES AND DROPS

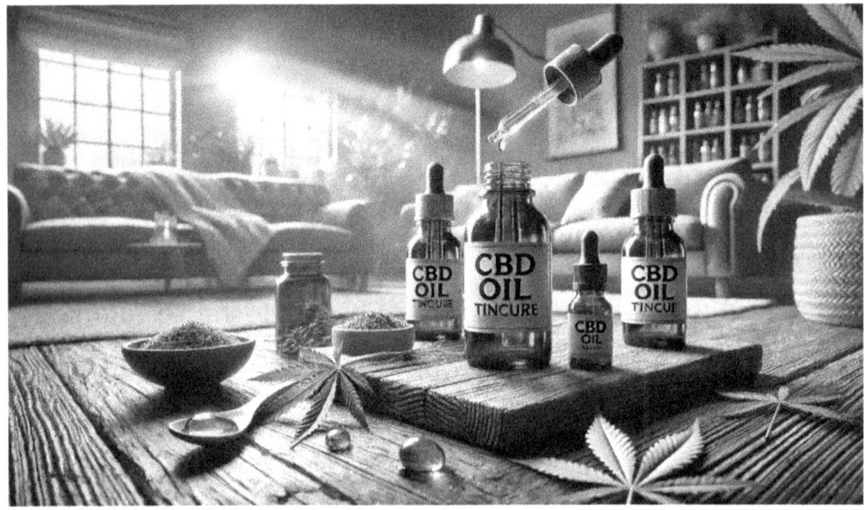

Getting CBD as a tincture or in drop form tends to be the most popular among users because they are the most versatile and easy to use of CBD products. You can get them in a range of concentrations and strains. For example, you can find Charlotte's Web tinctures available in concentrations that range from 250 milligrams to 500 milligrams.

Then there are Tasty Drops available in a range of flavors and concentrations from 150 milligrams to 300 milligrams. Tincture form allows you to simply place a few drops under your tongue so your body can absorb them and take them into your bloodstream. Some popular flavors among users include cinnamon, vanilla, and peppermint.

CBD OIL CONCENTRATES

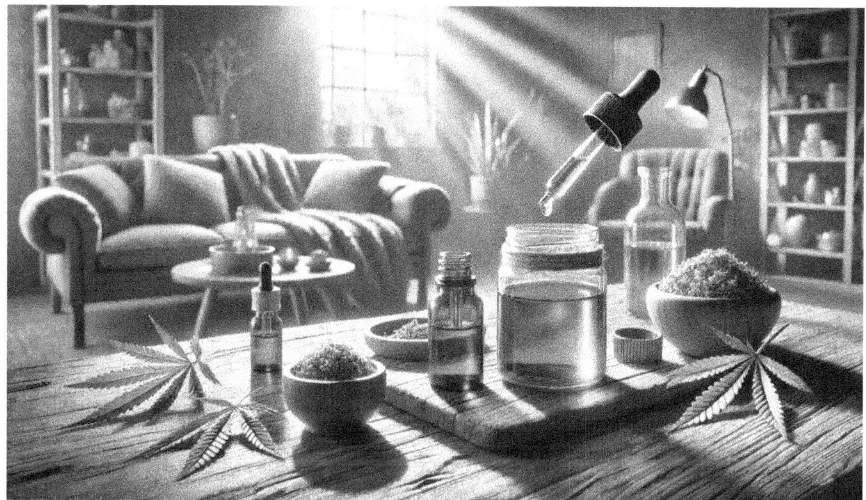

Those who typically choose CBD oil concentrates want a stronger form of CBD oil and are often the most concentrated. They typically have no added flavor and come as pure oil or wax crumbles. You can typically take them orally or use them with a vaporizer.

There is a wide variety of CBD oil concentrates to meet the needs of all users. However, for beginning CBD users, the concentrates can be a little strong. Concentrates are best for those who need a stronger form of CBD, either later in the disease process or as their body becomes more adjusted to using CBD.

CBD Vape-Oil in Vaporizers

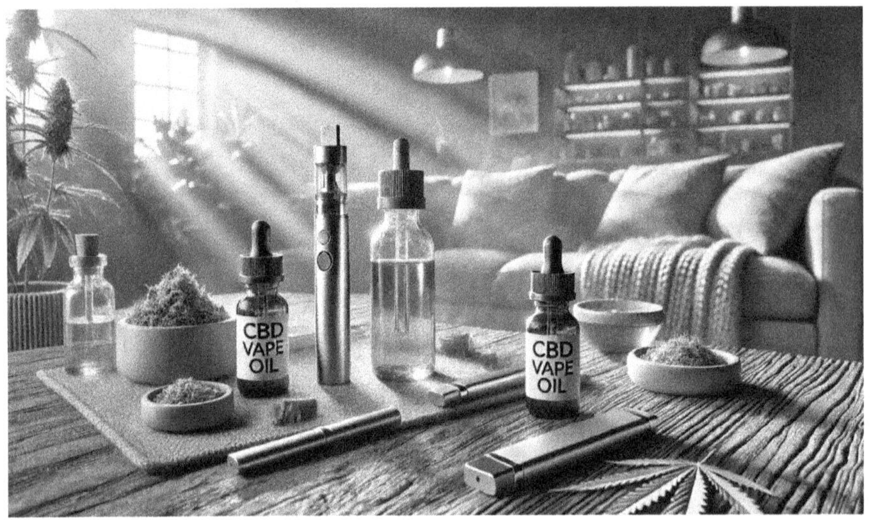

Vaporizers are devices that work basically the same as an e-pen. You use concentrated CBD vape oil in a vaporizer, and as the oil vaporizes, it is inhaled into the lungs and absorbed into the bloodstream. This is the fastest way to take CBD oil so it takes effect more quickly in your body for fast pain relief.

There are a number of vape oil options when it comes to CBD, and you can often find vaporizer kits to help you get started. You can find CBD vape oils with and without terpenes, as well as a number of unusual flavors for those who want to try something a little different. You can also get CBD vape oil in a range of concentrations to fit any type of pain level.

If you are into vaping instead of consuming CBD in other forms, I highly recommend you read this book, "Weed This Way" by Nathan Farley. He has done an outstanding job explaining the vaping process and various devices you can use to consume various forms of marijuana-related products.

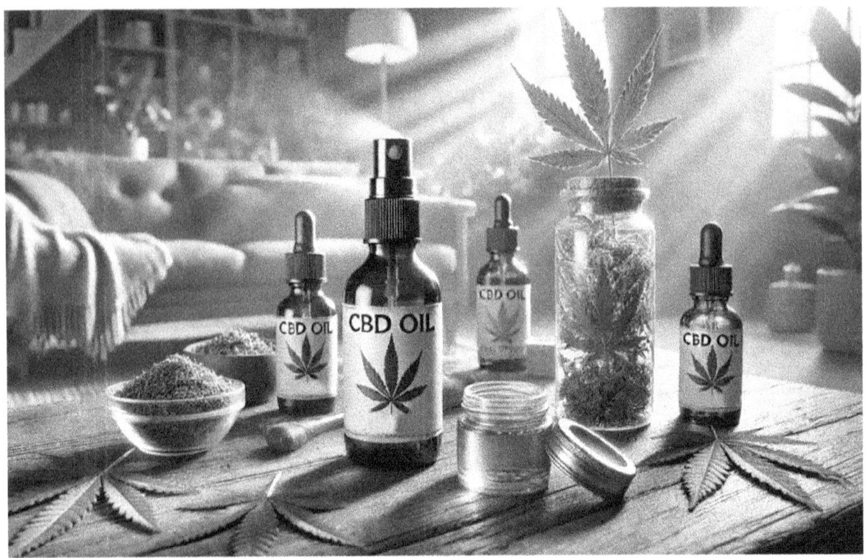

Oral sprays have the fewest flavor options. However, this option is often found mixed with hemp oil, so you get the benefits of both hemp oil and CBD oil in an easy-to-administer format. These options also allow you to have more CBD than a drop or tincture form.

Make sure you choose oral sprays that feature non-GMO hemp with no pesticides, herbicides or chemical fertilizers. Often, your flavor options are original, vanilla, and peppermint, with concentrations up to 500 milligrams. It is often suggested to apply two sprays under the tongue, hold for 30 seconds, and repeat twice a day to start.

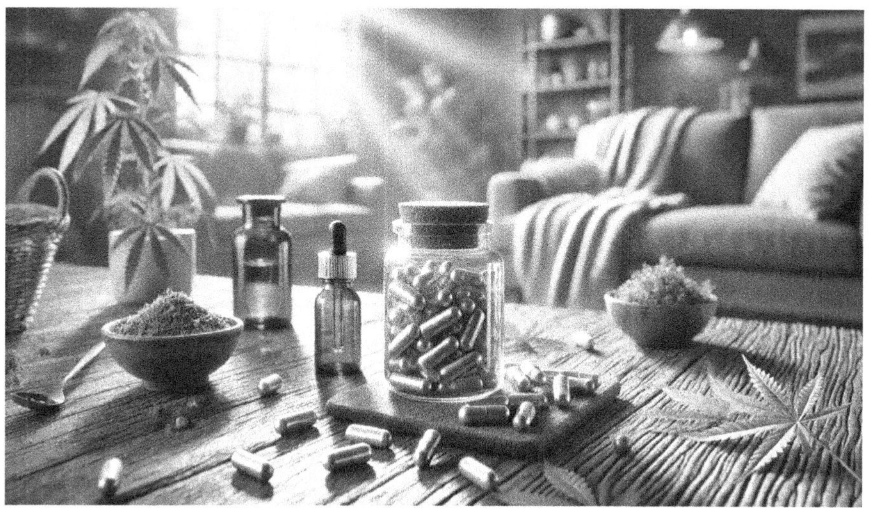

CBD in capsule form is available from a range of brands. You can get oil capsules mixed with hemp oil or standard capsules with powdered CBD. You can even find a soft gel version of CBD that you can take as a suppository for those who may have trouble swallowing a pill. The capsule forms are easily dissolvable and are quickly digested, so they can be absorbed by the body quickly.

Capsules give you the biggest range of concentrations when it comes to taking CBD and are best for those who want to keep track of their daily CBD intake in a measured form. You can also take them easily, so you can take the medication with you to work or while traveling. It also makes it easy to gradually increase your dose until you reach your ideal dose.

CBD EDIBLES

CBD also comes in a range of edible options. You can find them added to honey, peanut butter, and even a caffeine chew. You can find them in a number of flavors, such as cinnamon, citrus, mint, and sour apple, in a convenient daily chew format. They come with and without hemp oil.

You are sure to find a strength and format that makes it easy to add CBD to your daily diet. You can find strengths ranging from 5-milligram chews up to 500-milligram honey and peanut butter forms. Edibles can be added to your daily meals or taken as a snack between meals to help you get through the day.

CBD OIL-BASED LOTIONS AND BALMS

CBD oil can be added to a range of creams, lotions, and balms for immediate topical pain relief. This allows you to target your relief to where the pain is with high-quality CBD extract. Make sure you choose products that feature CBD extracted from organic cannabis plants for the most potent effect.

You can choose scented topicals to suit your preference, or get unscented versions for those sensitive to smells. You can also get them in a range of concentrations to suit your needs, such as for joint pain relief.

4 POPULAR CBD OIL EXTRACTION METHODS

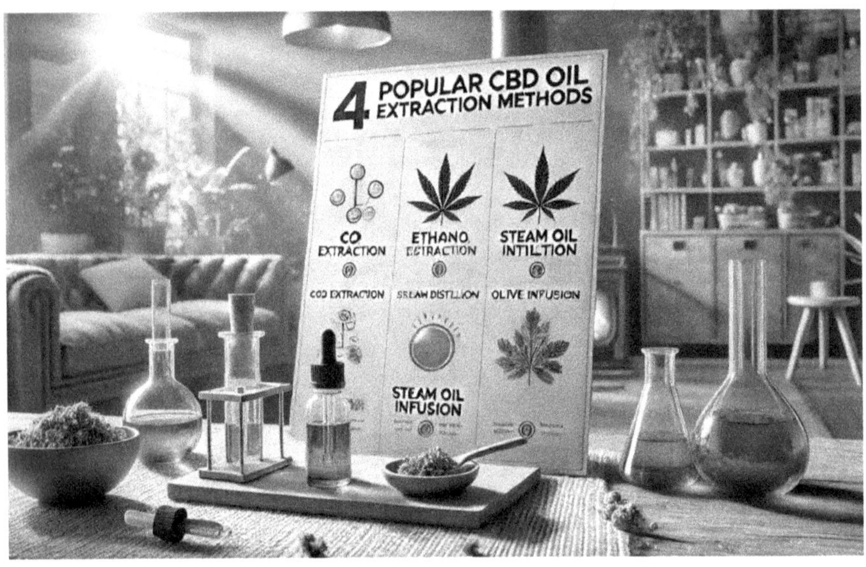

The goal of CBD extraction is quite simple: you want to pull the cannabinoid out and have it in a highly concentrated form. This makes it suitable for human consumption. To extract the oil you are seeking, you have to use a plant rich in CBD.

There are special strains, such as Charlotte's Web, that have a high level of CBD concentration as well as a low THC concentration. You need a favorable CBD/THC ratio. So that because if plants have a THC concentration of even

6%, the extra high CBD content should hopefully yield no THC effects.

There are various strains of industrial hemp. This is another way to extract CBD. They are grown legally around the world. Fedora 17 is one of the more popular industrial hemp strains. This is because it is extremely low in THC content.

So this means that any CBD extracted from it will have basically no psychoactive effects. CBD oil that is made from hemp is completely legal in virtually every country around the world and all 50 states in the U.S. This is due to the lack of THC content.

There are many methods for extracting CBD oil. Some are better for home use than others. It is essential to be very safe, no matter the method you choose. Here are the four most common methods for extracting CBD oil.

THE CO2 CANNABIS EXTRACTION METHOD

This method of CBD extraction is divided into three categories: supercritical, subcritical and 'mid-critical.' However, supercritical is the most commonly used. It is the most commonly used extraction method because it is safe to perform at home and yields a pure product.

This method uses pressurized carbon dioxide to pull CBD from the plant. CO_2 acts like a solvent. This method is safe and effective, but the equipment to use it is very expensive. You would need sophisticated machines used to freeze the CO_2 gas, then compress it into a cold liquid state

Now that you have liquid CO_2, you need to increase the temperature and pressure beyond the point at which it becomes 'supercritical.' This term means that CO_2 can now adopt properties that are halfway between those of a gas and a liquid simultaneously.

Effectively, supercritical CO_2 can fill a container (like a gas) while maintaining density (like a liquid). When CO_2 is in its supercritical state, it is ideal for chemical extraction because it won't cause denaturation or other damage that would render it unfit for human consumption.

To extract CBD oil using this technique, you begin with liquid CO_2 and increase its pressure with a compressor. You must also raise its temperature using a heater. The next step involves passing the supercritical carbon dioxide through some high-quality cannabis, which should be in an extractor. Now, CO2 will extract the essential oils from the plant.

There are several benefits to using CO2. Safety is the first benefit because CO2 is a common food additive used to produce things like carbonated soft drinks. CO2 is actually very effective; it has been used as an extraction solvent for many years. Common uses include extracting caffeine from coffee and producing essential oils. CO2 is an effective method for keeping your final product pure. There are fewer risks for contaminants with this method.

Just like there are benefits, there are some definite drawbacks to this method. It is very expensive. If you had to purchase all of this equipment outright, it would cost you about $40,000. You also need the technical ability and the 'know-how' to actually carry out the extraction. This is absolutely not a method for amateurs.

This is a complex method that, for most, should be studied exclusively for educational purposes. This video can show you the whole process.

https://www.youtube.com/watch?v=dgfPI0MbLho

THE OLIVE OIL EXTRACTION METHOD

This is the most beginner-friendly method for CBD extraction. Other liquids can be used, but olive oil is by far the most common in this type of extraction. This method is perfect for those who want to do CBD oil extraction at home.

The first step is to ensure the raw plant material is at the right temperature. This means you have to heat your plant to a specific temperature for a set period to activate its chemicals.

You want to heat your plant to 284 degrees Fahrenheit for half an hour. Then add the plant material to the olive oil and heat to 212 degrees Fahrenheit for up to 2 hours. This process will extract the oil you want.

The olive oil extraction method is very safe, so you won't have to worry about blowing anything up or setting things on fire. It is also very inexpensive. You most likely won't have to buy anything that's not already in your kitchen.

However, this extraction method yields a *perishable* product. So as soon as it is done, make sure to put it in a cool, dark place as quickly as possible. This method also yields very little oil, so it would be a poor choice for companies but a good one for personal use.

Here's a video of how olive oil extraction works:

https://www.youtube.com/watch?v=aieNV3V4b_s

THE DRY ICE EXTRACTION METHOD

The dry ice extraction method is another CBD extraction technique that can be performed at home. This method does take more time and effort than oil extraction. Here is what you need to gather.

- 3 pounds of dry ice.

- A mirror

- A paint scraper

- Thick heat-resistant gloves and eye protection.

- 5-gallon plastic bucket, clear

- 3 bubble hash mesh bags: 73, 160 and 220 microns.

- 3 large glass jars to use as storage.

Put on your gloves and chosen eye protection, then chop up the cannabis plant into small chunks and place it in the bucket. Make sure to cover the chunks with dry ice, then leave them for 3 minutes; try to fill the bucket only halfway. This will result in the freezing of the trichome resins. Next, place the 73-micron bag over the bucket and shake for 4 minutes to knock the frozen trichomes off.

Turn the bucket upside down over the mirror, then shake as much resin as possible through the mesh bag. Next, scrape the hash off the mirror with your scraper and place it into one of the jars. Repeat with the 160 and 220-micron mesh bags; this will give you three distinct strains.

This method is a little involved but easily doable. It will also leave very little in the mess department. You will get a much higher yield than with oil extraction. However, if you accidentally shake it for too long, you could end up with a lower-quality product. Ordering online is pretty much the only option for getting those three pounds of dry ice.

This method has to be carried out with great care. Following along with this video to help you as you go.

THE SOLVENT EXTRACTION METHOD

This is the method typically used for small-scale CBD oil production due to its low cost, readily available equipment, and simple process.

Some typical solvents include butane, grain alcohol, isopropyl alcohol, hexane or ethanol. Some do consider this process dangerous due to the use of highly flammable solvents such as butane and various alcohols. I personally do not recommend using solvents such as butane or pure grain alcohol.

Using such a highly flammable solvent can destroy some of the therapeutic plant waxes and decrease the medicinal value of the CBD oil. But there is a much safer and truly efficient way to do this if you follow a simple yet precise procedure. In this process, I use ethanol and not butane or any pure grain alcohol. Once you read the procedure and watch the video, you will know why I say it is simple and easy to follow.

<u>**To do this properly, you need the followings:**</u>

1 Drip Coffee Maker

Few Coffee filter papers

1 lighter

2 Small glass bowls

1 Large glass bowl

1 large plastic spoon

1 fine strainer

16 oz. bottle of isopropyl alcohol or Ethanol (60% pure)

1 oz. Bag of Dry Cannabis

1 Home water distiller machine

<u>**Process:**</u>

Mix dry cannabis with alcohol in a large glass bowl. Mix thoroughly with a plastic spoon. Let it soak for a few minutes. Then use the strainer to separate the liquid from the solid. Next, put a paper coffee filter inside the coffee maker (don't turn the coffee maker on, just let it drip) and pour the liquid so you can separate the fine dust of cannabis from the liquid. Once you have the liquid, use a water distiller to separate the ethanol from the oil.

Once the oil is separated, pour it into a small glass bowl and put it on the coffee pot warmer and turn the coffee maker on so the glass bowl can heat up and let the tiny ethanol particles evaporate. Leave it on there for a few hours. The end product should be a dark brownish-looking, thick, oily substance that is 100% pure CBD oil.

Just to make sure there is no ethanol left in there, dip a paperclip into the liquid, then try to light it with a lighter. If it catches fire, leave it on the coffee pot warmer for a few more hours.

Here is a clear YouTube video of how it is done, take a look

http://tinyurl.com/CBDOIL-Extraction

It is only appropriate for some situations, but using high-grade alcohol will yield a higher-grade product. This is also a pretty straightforward process: once you have the equipment, it works simply. However, since both butane and ethanol are highly flammable, you should take appropriate safety measures before trying this method.

Before we move on to how you can take CBD oil, let me touch on something that has been coming up on everyone's radar frequently.

SYNTHETIC VS. WHOLE PLANT FOR CBD OIL

When making CBD oil, one of the most important considerations is whether to use synthetic or whole-plant CBD. Let's consider which option is best.

Quite simply, a February 2015 article published in the journal *Pharmacology and Pharmacy* discussed a study from Israel that documented the superior therapeutic properties of the whole plant CBD cannabis extract when compared to synthetic, single-molecule Cannabidiol.

The study found that the administration of pure, single-molecule CBD had a bell-shaped dose-response curve. This means that once the amount of CBD reached a certain point, the therapeutic effect declined significantly. This is a characteristic of all single-molecule CBD, manifested as bell-shaped dose responses. It poses a serious obstacle that limits the usefulness of CBD oil in a clinical context.

In tests comparing both types of CBD oil, the results confirmed the findings of preclinical research. A different dose-response pattern was observed with whole-plant CBD oil.

The whole-plant CBD-rich oil extract showed direct, dose-dependent inhibition. Also, the testing found that a small amount of whole-plant CBD was needed to achieve positive effects, whereas a larger amount of synthetic CBD was required for the same effects.

So, in a nutshell, it is very clear that if you are looking for clean, potent, and naturally rich CBD oil, it is best to go with whole-plant CBD rather than synthetic ones.

How to Take CBD

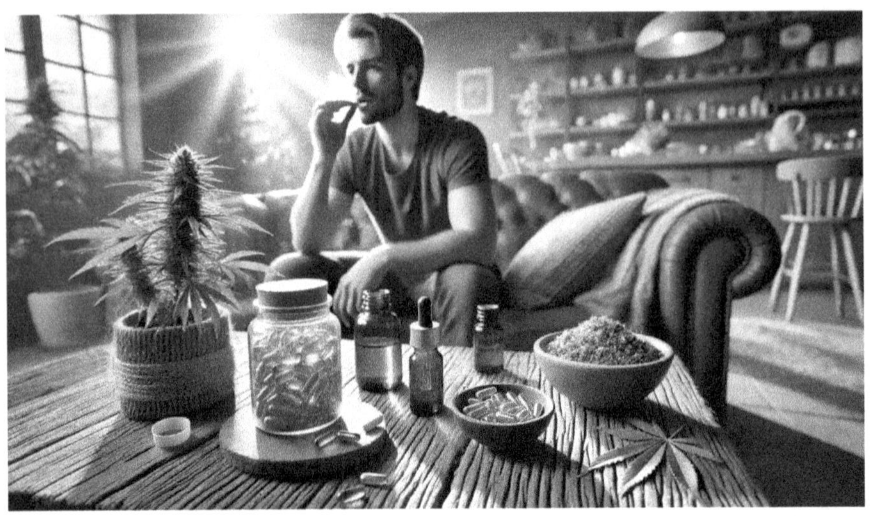

With all the forms of CBD available, you will likely find yourself asking what the best way to use CBD is. You can find it in a range of forms, including tinctures, vaping oils, sprays, edibles, and topicals, so you are sure to find one that meets your individual needs. The main idea behind taking CBD is to make sure you choose a method that gets the cannabinoids into your body easily so you can get the results you want.

This means that when choosing the right way to take CBD, you need to think about your optimal dose, the results you want to get from taking CBD and how long you want the pain relief to last. Therefore, there is no general rule when it comes to taking CBD products. Contrary to popular belief, most people prefer not to smoke their CBD, although vaping is becoming a popular option for alleviating pain symptoms quickly and for effects that can sometimes last up to a few hours.

Often, taking CBD orally allows the effects to last longer than just a few hours; however, it takes longer to take effect, ranging from 10 minutes to over an hour and a half after administration. So again, it comes down to a preference for the desired effect.

Another popular way is through tinctures, taken by dropping a couple of drops on or under your tongue. This dosage ranges from 100mg to 1000mg. They are the most common usage of CBD available on the market. For this method to be most effective, make sure you do not swallow the liquid right away. Instead, you want to ingest as much as you can before actually swallowing it. To do this, put the drops under your tongue and on the sides of your cheeks as long as you can before swallowing.

The use of capsules is another method. CBD capsules are great to add CBD to your daily diet as a supplement. This method is much easier to take than tinctures. These capsules' dosage typically range 10 to 25mg of CBD. Taking them is simple. Just have one or two capsules daily with water.

 CBD concentrates usually have the strongest dosage of CBD when compared to other CBD products. They can contain more than 10 times the amount found in the average CBD product. They are also very convenient.

They only take a few seconds to consume. For this reason, CBD concentrates are seen to be more popular with customers who are extremely busy but need a high-potency CBD. Concentrates are taken similarly to tinctures, without the need to wait before fully digesting them.

CBD sprays are typically the weakest in concentration among CBD products. The typical concentration of CBD sprays ranges from 1-3mg.

As I just mentioned, you can always use vape oil. To use CBD vape oil, you will need an e-cigarette, vape pen, or vaporizer. Add heat and inhale the appropriate amount of vape oil into your choice of device

CBD strips are a simple way to administer medicine to your body. The dissolvable CBD strips don't require an injection. They don't need to be digested. And they don't carry with them the risk of causing stomach problems. CBD strips are a simple yet effective way to get the medicine you need.

Always consult a physician before you take any CBD product for medicinal purposes. It can also be beneficial to talk to the budtenders at your local dispensary. They can provide useful information as well.

As for dosage, I always recommend starting small and increasing it slowly once you see how you react. As a general rule, start with the lowest possible dose and maintain it for 3 days. This will give your body time to react. Once you know how you feel at a certain dosage, you can adjust up or down for the next three days. If you feel any discomfort, decrease your dosage.

There are topical options for those who don't wish to take CBD oil with these methods. There are many topical options available, such as lotions and lip balms, which are known to help with acute symptoms like pain and inflammation, skin care, psoriasis, and cancer treatment symptoms, as well as aging-related concerns like wrinkles.

CBD topicals are to be used just like their non-CBD counterparts. You would use them whenever you deem necessary. They can also be used for skin conditions. Simply apply generously to areas of the body that could benefit from it.

RECIPES – DESSERT, SKINCARE & OINTMENT

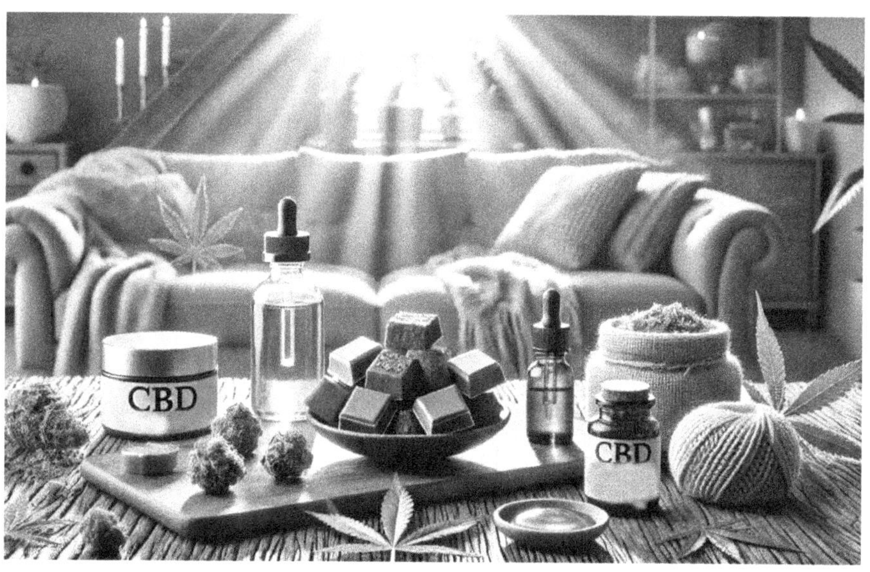

GREAT FOOD AND DESSERT RECIPES

For those who want to take their CBD orally but have a difficult time with the taste of CBD oil or using methods to do so, there are some great options. Choosing to bake with your CBD oil will not affect its potency and will result in a very palatable way to take your CBD oil.

Here are some quick and easy recipes anyone can make.

Brownie Recipe Infused with CBD Vegetable Oil

This is a simple brownie recipe that uses CBD oil instead of your typical vegetable oil. Most people will have these ingredients, and already have them in their kitchen. You can also mix it up by adding chopped nuts, chocolate chips, or even fruit to make your CBD-infused brownies even more special (and enjoyable!).

Ingredients:

1 Cup of oil

1 gram of 99% CBD Isolate

1 Cup sugar

1 teaspoon vanilla

2 eggs

¼ teaspoon baking powder

1/3 Cup cocoa powder

¼ teaspoon salt

½ Cup flour.

Direction:

1.   Preheat oven to 350°F.

2.   Mix the CBD Isolate with the oil. Mix oil and sugar until well blended.

3.   Add eggs and vanilla. Then stir until completely blended.

4.   Mix all of your dry ingredients in a separate bowl.

5. Slowly stir the dry ingredients into the liquid mixture.

6.   Pour the entire contents of your bowl into a greased 9×9 square pan.

7.   Bake for 20 minutes or until all the sides start to pull away from the pan. Cool completely before cutting. The resulting brownies will contain 24.75mg of CBD if cut into 9 pieces.

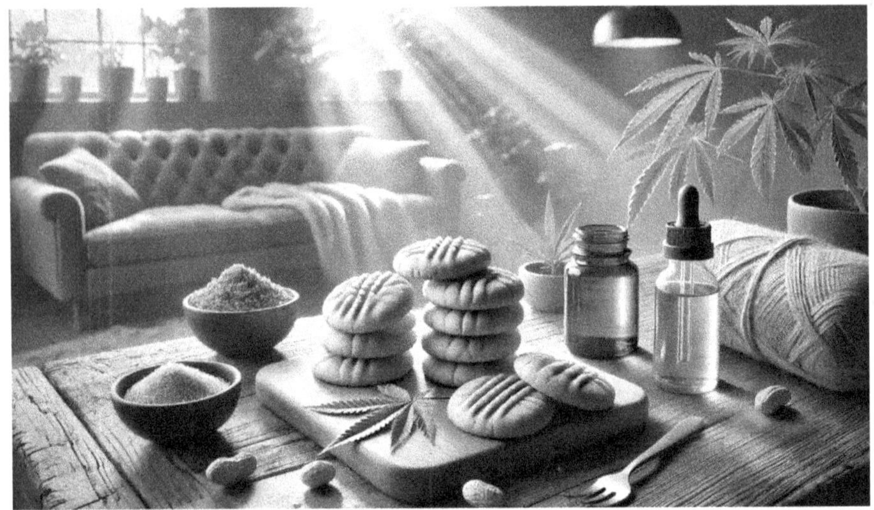

These cookies are plain delicious. They are the perfect way to replace your daily CBD. This recipe will make about three dozen cookies, each with about 28 mg of CBD. These cookies use coconut oil instead of butter. This makes them a bit healthier and a perfect recipe to mix in your CBD oil.

<u>Here's what you need:</u>

1 ½ Cup of creamy peanut butter

1 Cup coconut oil, softened

1 gram of 99% CBD Isolate

2 Cups light brown sugar, packed

2 large eggs

2 Tablespoons vanilla extract

2 Cups of flour

4 teaspoons of cornstarch

2 teaspoons of baking soda

½ teaspoon of salt

<u>Here's what you'll do:</u>

1. Combine the 1 gram of 99% CBD Isolate with the coconut oil

In a stand mixer, combine peanut butter, coconut oil mixture, eggs, and sugar

2. On Medium-High speed, cream mixture until light and fluffy

Make sure to scrape the sides of the bowl. Then add vanilla and beat for an additional minute

3. Then add flour, cornstarch, baking soda, and salt. Just mix for another minute

4. Use a cookie scoop to form mounds and place dough mounds on a large plate. Then cover the tray with plastic wrap and refrigerate for 2 hours. When ready to cook, leave the dough out for 15-20 minutes to warm up slightly for the best results.

5. Preheat oven to 350 degrees. Place the dough on a lined baking sheet, leaving 2 inches between them.

6. Bake for 7-9 minutes or until tops are just set.

7. Finally, allow cookies to cool on the baking sheet for 10 minutes.

You can store cookies in an airtight container for up to 1 week or in the freezer for up to 3 months. You can also store the uncooked dough in your freezer for up to 3 months.

CBD INFUSED PEANUT BRITTLE RECIPE

If you are not into baked goods, this one is for you. You can definitely never beat a classic! Take an old-fashioned recipe and turn it into an infusion recipe! This recipe is simple to make and very fun! Everyone loves peanut brittle! Here is a quick, easy way to infuse CBD into your favorite childhood snack!

<u>Here's what you need:</u>

1/4 Cup of water

1 Cup of sugar

1/2 Cup light corn syrup

1/4 teaspoon salt

1 Cup of chopped peanuts

1 teaspoon of baking soda

4 ½ Tablespoons of oil

¼ gram of CBD isolate

<u>Here's what you'll do:</u>

1. Using a Double Boiler, bring your oil of choice to a boil and stir frequently

2. Remove from heat when sugar completely dissolves

3. Add the Infused Isolate and add 1 Teaspoon of Baking Soda

4. Mix vigorously

5. Pour into a greased baking sheet or Pyrex

6. You can add some optional Chocolate Chips or Berries once your brittle has slightly cooled and mix lightly.

7. Lay flat and let cool for about an hour

8. Break and serve!

CHOCOLATE CHIP COOKIES

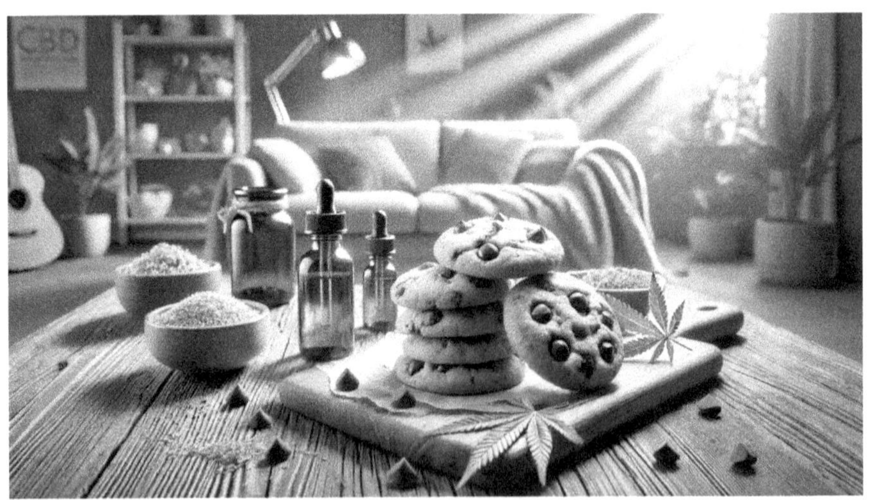

Like peanut brittle, these cookies will take you back to childhood. They are warm and gooey and filled with chocolate chips- just the way they should be.

<u>Here's what you'll need.</u>

⅔ cup liquid Cannabis Coconut Oil

1 1/4 cup coconut sugar

½ cup almond milk, unsweetened

2 tablespoons spring water

1 tablespoon arrowroot starch

1 teaspoon vanilla extract

2 cups gluten-free all-purpose flour

1 cup vegan chocolate chips

⅔ cup raw organic cocoa powder

1 teaspoon baking soda

½ teaspoon sea salt

<u>**Here's what you'll do:**</u>

1. Preheat oven to 375 degrees. Grease a baking sheet.

2. Mix Cannabis Coconut Oil, sugar, almond milk, brown sugar, water, arrowroot starch and vanilla extract in a large bowl. Set aside.

3. Mix flour, vegan chocolate chips, cocoa powder, baking soda, and salt in a separate bowl.

4. Add the flour mixture to the oil mixture slowly. Stir all ingredients together.

5. Form dough into 1-inch balls and place them two inches apart on a baking sheet.

6. Bake in preheated oven for 10 minutes.

7. Remove cookies from the oven. Leave on baking sheet for 5 minutes.

8. Transfer cookies to a wire rack to cool before serving.

Raw Chocolate CBD Oil Macaroons

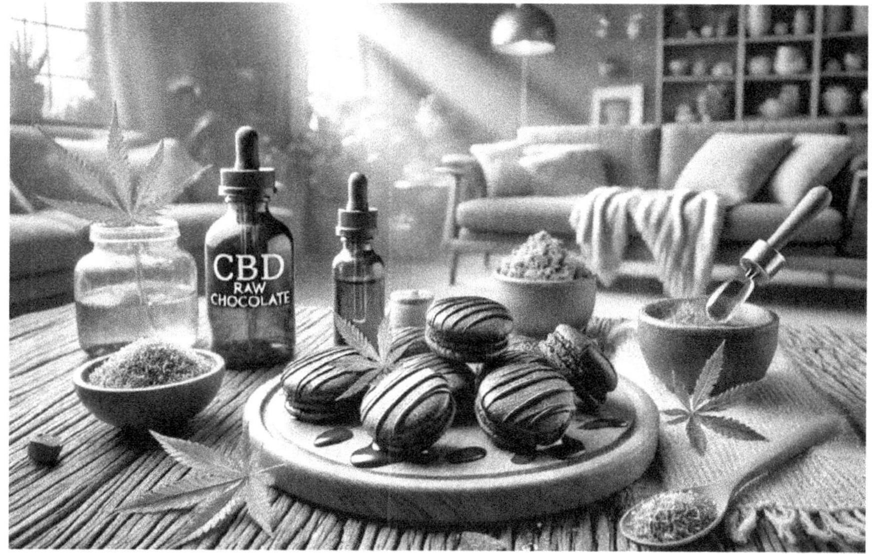

Chocolate hemp macaroons are chewy and chocolaty with a definite hemp flavor. To make these delicious hemp oil-infused macarons, you'll only need a few things to whip these up.

Here's what you'll need:

3 tablespoons melted Cacao Butter

3 tablespoons melted Coconut Crème

3 tablespoons Hemp Butter

3 tablespoons warm water

1 ½ cups shredded coconut

5 tablespoons cacao powder

3 tablespoons xylitol

7-8 drops stevia

2 pinches of salt

In a double boiler or a bowl set in hot water, whisk the cacao butter, coconut crème, hemp butter, water, xylitol, stevia, and salt. Sift the cacao powder in, then stir in the shredded coconut until all ingredients are evenly combined. Use a mini ice cream scoop to make balls, transferring them to a parchment paper-lined tray. Chill in the fridge for at least 4 hours, until firm. Store in the fridge for up to 7 days.

CBD CARROT CAKE

2 cups all-purpose flour

1 teaspoon baking soda

2 teaspoons cinnamon

1/4 teaspoon salt

3 eggs

3/4 cup buttermilk

1 cup Hemp Oil

1 1/2 cups sugar

2 teaspoons vanilla

2 1/2 cups shredded carrots

1 cup flaked coconut

1 cup chopped walnuts

1 cup raisins

Frosting

1/2 cup butter softened (or CBD Butter)

1 cup cream cheese

4 cups powdered sugar

1 teaspoon vanilla extract

<u>Here's what you'll do:</u>

1. **Preheat** oven to **350 degrees**.

2. Sift together flour, baking soda, salt and cinnamon in a medium-sized bowl. Set aside.

3. Combine eggs, buttermilk, CBD oil & Vegetable Oil mix, sugar and vanilla in a separate bowl. Mix well.

4. Add the flour mixture to the Oil mixture. Stir well.

5. Combine shredded carrots, coconut, walnuts, and raisins in a separate bowl.

6. Add carrot mixture to batter and mix thoroughly.

7. Pour batter into pan and bake for 1 hour, or until toothpick comes out clean.

8. Remove cake from oven and let cool.

9. While cake is cooling – In a medium bowl, combine butter, cream cheese, powdered sugar and 1

teaspoon vanilla to make the frosting. Beat until the mixture is smooth and creamy.

10. Frost cake with icing. Store in refrigerator.

11. Cut and serve.

12.

STRAWBERRY SMOOTHIE

This smoothie is healthy and delicious. You only need a few ingredients, and it is very simple to make and takes very little time. The chia gel does need about twenty minutes to set, but other than that, this smoothie is a snap to make.

Here's what you'll need:

3 Tbsp. Organic Virgin Coconut Oil

2 Tbsp. Organic Chia Seeds made into Chia Gel –(¼ C. chia seeds to 1 ¼ C warm water- let sit at least 20 minutes)

2 Tbsp. Organic Hemp seed

1 Tbsp. Organic Hemp Oil

6 strawberries Organic, frozen.

1 Tbsp. honey

2 cups of almond milk

<u>Here's what you'll do</u>

1. Mix Chia Gel, take a shower. After showering and getting ready for your day, grab your blender. Throw in the ingredients above, in no specific order.

2. Let blend for a good 3 minutes or more.

3. Pour into your favorite breakfast glass and enjoy.

You will have energy and be satisfied beyond lunchtime. Makes it easy to eat, good for a light and healthy lunch!

SKINCARE RECIPES

Hemp oil is also great for the skin. Here are some great homemade topical remedies that can help soothe many common skin concerns.

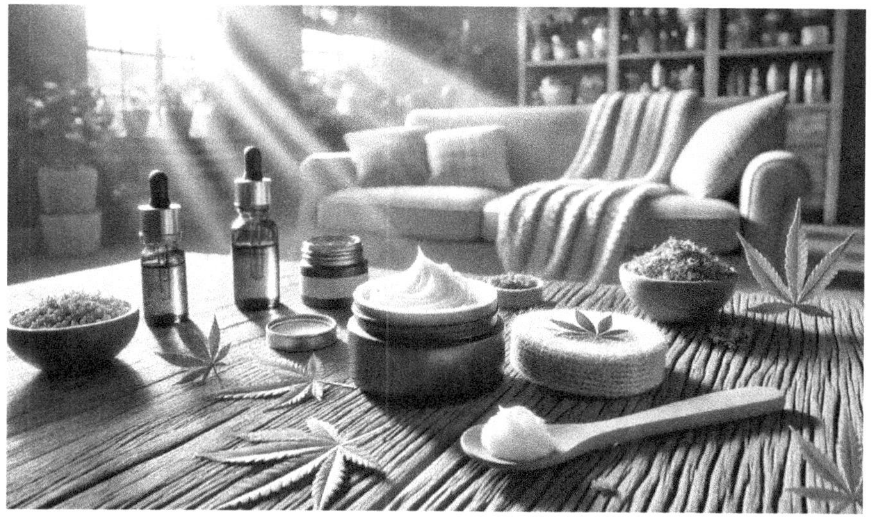

This shea butter balm is amazing for dry skin and for those with eczema. It is soothing and cooling. It can be used every day as much as needed,

To create your topical shea butter balm, you'll need the following:

1 1/2 teaspoon CBD Oil

1 1/2 teaspoon grated beeswax

1 1/2 teaspoon shea butter

10 drops of essential oil of your choice

1. Melt beeswax and Shea butter in a microwave-safe bowl for about one minute. Stir in CBD oil and essential oils

2. Pour into the desired container and allow to set.

Once hardened, your homemade DIY CBD hemp topical is ready to use and can be massaged into the skin, muscles, and joints for desired effects.

MAGNESIUM BODY BUTTER

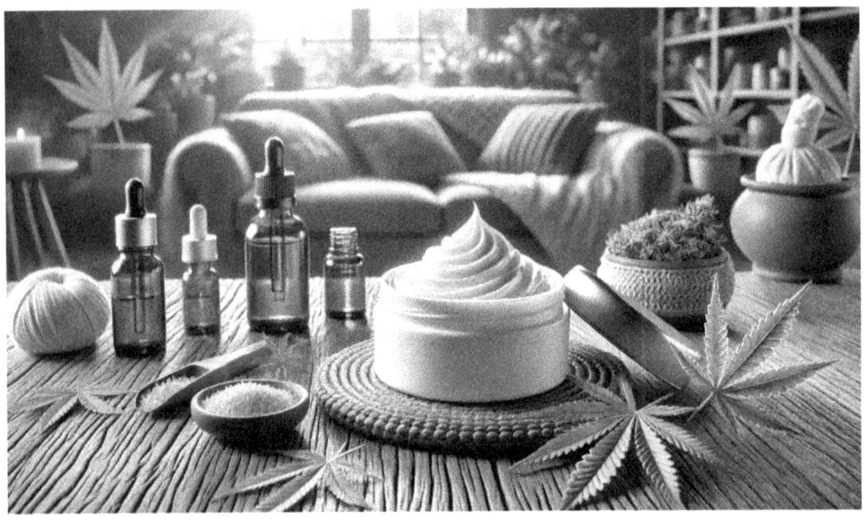

This body butter is the best for relaxation! Adding essential oils makes the body butter smell amazing, and then you get the additional benefits from the properties of the essential oils.

To create your CBD-infused magnesium body butter, you'll need:

½ cup cocoa butter

½ cup coconut oil

¼ cup magnesium oil

10 drops of essential oil, like lavender, eucalyptus, or peppermint

The desired amount of CBD Oil

1. Melt the coconut oil and cocoa butter together over medium heat.

2. Add magnesium oil, your chosen essential oil, and CBD liquid.

3. Stir the mixture and allow it to cool.

4. After the mix has cooled, begin to whip into a body butter. Using a hand mixer will help you achieve a light and fluffy finished product. Store your homemade body butter in an airtight container.

For this, you will need a ½ ounce of CBD high cannabis strain and ½ cup of shea butter, coconut oil or beeswax. You can even choose to use a combination of the three, since this gives you additional benefits and is often highly recommended. With these ingredients, you can use the following steps to make a CBD ointment for topical pain relief.

1. Place the oils in a glass or ceramic mixing bowl. When using a combination of the three, use a wooden spoon and make sure they are mixed well.
2. Place a large pot on the stove and fill it halfway or less with water.
3. Once the water is hot, but not boiling, then you can place the mixing bowl in the pot. Be careful to make sure no water gets into the bowl.
4. Once the oils are liquefied and well blended, you can add the cannabis.
5. Allow everything to gently simmer while stirring every few minutes for at least 45 minutes. The longer the mixture simmers, the more potent the resulting ointment will be.

6. Strain the ointment through a cheesecloth into a glass container. Squeeze the cloth to make sure you get out every drop possible from the cannabis.

7. Allow the ointment mixture to cool completely before you use it.

8. After it is completely cool, you can use a spoon or spatula to move the ointment into a different container if you want.

9. Store the ointment in a cool, dark place, and it will be good for about two months.

A valuable tip is that if you make your ointment with beeswax or a beeswax-based combination, it will result in a firmer, more stable ointment.

An ointment made with CBD oil has the anti-inflammatory and anti-spasmodic properties of CBD, so it can reduce pain, enhance circulation, and promote cellular regeneration. There are a number of painful conditions that can be helped with CBD ointment, some of the most common ones are the following:

- ❖ Skin Conditions such as:
  - ➤ Eczema
  - ➤ Dermatitis

> - Psoriasis

> - Rashes

> - Fungal Infections

> - Dry Skin

> - Blisters

- Joint Pain

- Arthritis Pain

- Muscle Soreness

- Sprains

- Mild Injuries

- Wounds

- Cuts

- Scrapes

- Bruises

- Chronic Pain

- Multiple Sclerosis

- Nerve Pain

- Sciatica

- Seizures

- Muscle Spasms

- Earaches

- Migraines

- Menstrual Cramps

- Hemorrhoids

❖ Anxiety

❖ Depression

❖ PTSD

Whether you purchase or make your own CBD, you will need to know how to dose and take it properly. Let's look at the various ways you can take your CBD and how to get proper dosing.

CBD OIL DOSAGE FOR SPECIFIC PAIN CONDITIONS

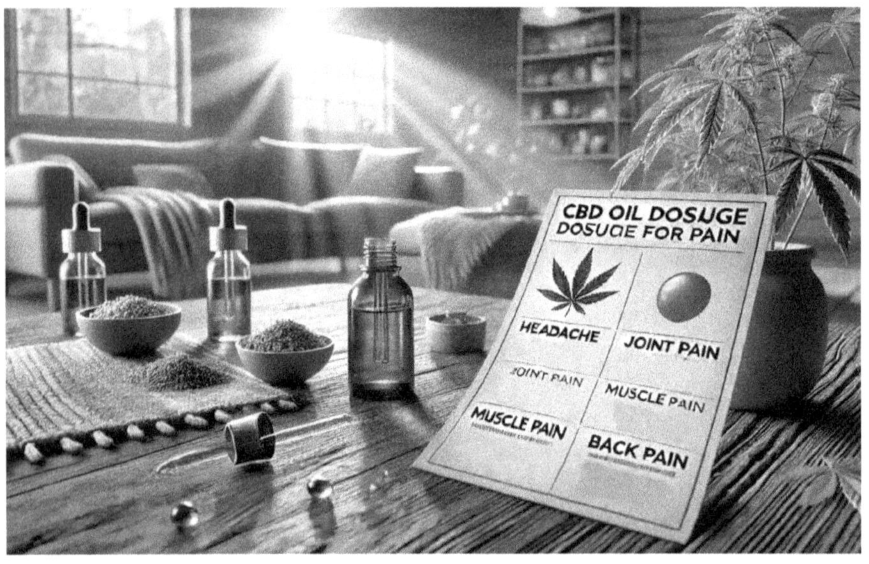

Chronic pain can manifest in a range of body areas, including muscles, organs, joints, body cavities, and ligaments. Pain can also be associated with a number of diseases and health conditions; most notably: ulcerative colitis, Crohn's disease, multiple sclerosis, Lyme disease, and fibromyalgia.

The chronic pain associated with these diseases can leave individuals functionless and even incapacitated. CBD oil provides not only pain relief but also helps support muscles, improve joint health, and enhance organ function.

The typical dosage of CBD oil is about 2.5 to 20 milligrams taken sublingually for 25 to 30 days. Use the following table to help you dose our CBD oil.

Pain Level	2-2 lbs.	26-45 lbs.	46-85 lbs.	86-150 lbs.	151-240 lbs.	241+ lbs.
Mild	4.5 mg	6 mg	9 mg	12 mg	18 mg	22.5 mg
Moderate	6 mg	9 mg	12 mg	15 mg	22.5 mg	30 mg
Severe	9 mg	12 mg	15 mg	18 mg	27 mg	45 mg

CBD oil is also a good choice for reducing pain since it provides your body with essential fatty acids. These fatty acids have the added benefit of helping your body to produce eicosanoids. Eicosanoids will help regulate bodily functions and keep body temperature and pain levels in balance.

Let's look at some specific dosing options for individual pain conditions that might require a little different dosing than the table above.

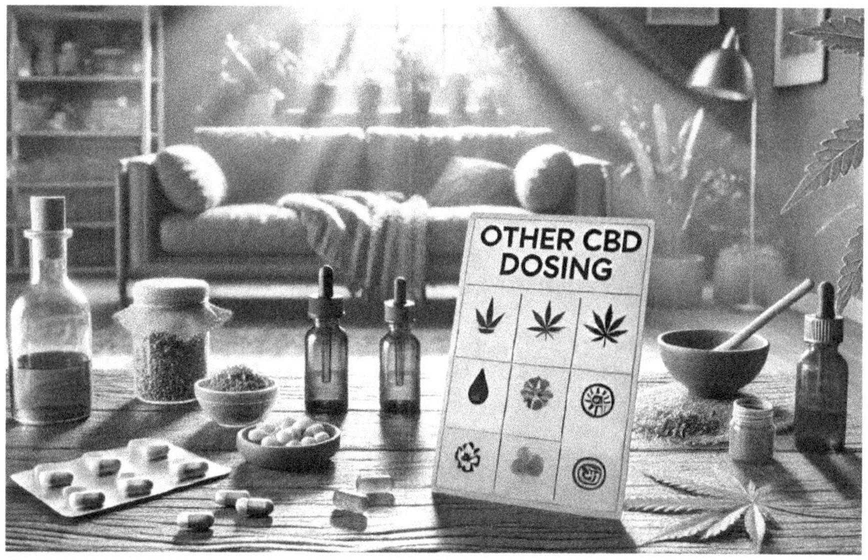

For those who have cancer, a major issue is a loss of appetite. To help with this, it is recommended to take 2.5 milligrams of THC orally with or without 1 milligram of CBD for a period of at least six weeks.

For those who have epilepsy, the recommended dose is 200 to 300 milligrams of CBD orally for at least four to five months.

For help treating any type of sleeping disorder, you can take 40 to 160 milligram CBD orally.

For treating symptoms associated with schizophrenia, you can take 40 to 1280 milligrams of CBD orally once a day for about four weeks.

For treating pain associated with glaucoma, you can place a single dose sublingually of about 20 to 40 milligrams. Dosages higher than this can result in increased eye pressure

NERVE PAIN AND NEUROPATHY

Both nerve pain and neuropathy can result in nerve damage. A number of conditions and factors can cause nerve pain and neuropathy, such as the following:

- Increased blood sugar
- Obesity
- Alcohol
- Diseases
- Vitamin deficiency
- Other conditions

Nerves are found throughout the body and brain. This means the pain can become very violent quickly, sometimes within an hour; plus, it can move around to different areas of the body.

For this type of pain, a good option is topical CBD oil. It is a good idea to mix it with wintergreen essential oil. Add about 30 to 35 drops of wintergreen essential oil to about 2 ounces (60 ml) of hemp oil. Apply a moderate amount of the oil to the affected area, then massage well and warm the area. Repeat this for a week or so to see if you get relief.

INFLAMMATION

CBD oil, when combined with essential oils and antioxidants, works together to reduce inflammation. Some good recipes for inflammation include the following:

Add 15 drops of Helichrysum and Cistus essential oils to one ounce or 30 ml of CBD oil. Blend well and apply to the inflamed area, repeating every few days for complete relief of pain associated with inflammation.

BACK PAIN

The nerves and muscles present in our back can result in a dull backache or the widespread pain that affects our everyday habits and routines. Our back muscles help us to lift weights and sit, stand and walk properly. A number of injuries and accidents can strain our back muscles. For back pain, consider the following recipe:

Combine one ounce or 30 ml of CBD oil with about ten to fifteen drops of birch and Frankincense essential oils. Mix well and apply several times a day to help reduce and relieve back pain.

MIGRAINES AND HEADACHES

Anyone who has ever experienced a headache or a migraine knows that it can affect just a part of the head or the whole head and can last from a few hours to a few days or more. Headaches can even cause such severe pain that, in some cases, they can cause disability. However, since headaches can be a sign of more serious medical conditions, it is important to talk to a doctor before trying the following recipe for headaches or migraines.

Start with about 10 ml of CBD oil and add about seven drops of grapefruit essential oil and three to four drops of peppermint essential oil. Apply a small amount to the back of your neck and/or temples and rub softly. It will help improve circulation and oxygenation while reducing inflammation and relieving the pain associated with headaches and migraines.

Joint Pain and Rheumatoid Arthritis

Rheumatoid arthritis and most other forms of joint pain are a type of autoimmune disorder. Autoimmune disorders can affect joints, skin, eyes, heart and blood vessels. In fact, when left untreated, autoimmune disorders can lead to bone deformity due to bone erosion. Help joint pain with the following recipe:

Start with a ratio of 2:1 or 3:1 Omega-6 to Omega-3. This will help suppress inflammation that typically occurs due to rheumatoid arthritis. Next, you'll want to add about 20 to 30 drops of birch and Frankincense essential oils to about 2 ounces (60 ml) of CBD oil. Apply this mixture on the painful area four to five times a week with a five-day break.

Varicose Veins

Varicose veins are found on the legs as a result of circulatory problems. Those who have suffered from this condition know how painful they are, and CBD oil can help with all of them. CBD oil helps relieve the heaviness, swelling, pain, and visible signs associated with enlarged veins in varicose veins. For relief, try the following recipe:

Start with about 1 ½ ounces (45 ml) of CBD oil and add 20 to 25 drops of Cypress and Immortelle essential oils. This mixture can help reduce the pain and appearance of varicose veins.

ANXIETY RELIEF

CBD can help you manage anxiety. Some researchers think it may actually change the way your brain's receptors respond to serotonin. Serotonin is a chemical that is linked to mental health. Your brain's receptors are these tiny proteins that are attached to your cells. They receive chemical signals, then work with your cells to respond to various stimuli.

CBD may help relieve anxiety in several ways. It can help reduce stress and eliminate anxiety symptoms, such as an increased heart rate. Those who have PTSD could have improved symptoms through the use of CBD. CBD oil can also help those with insomnia; it can slowly relax your mind and body, and eventually, you will fall asleep.

Many patients taking cannabis for anxiety, depression, spasms and pediatric seizure disorders find it is best to start with a moderate dose of CBD-dominant remedies, such as a CBD: THC ratio of more than 10:1. A low THC remedy, while not intoxicating, isn't often the best therapeutic dose. A combination of CBD and THC often has a greater therapeutic effect and covers a wider range of conditions than CBD or THC alone.

ANTI-SEIZURE

CBD has been considered a benefit to those who have epilepsy. Though research is still in its early days, CBD oil has been able to be able to reduce the number of seizures in some people with epilepsy.

NEUROPROTECTIVE

CBD could help people with neurodegenerative disorders. These are diseases that cause the brain and nerves to deteriorate over time. Here is a list of diseases for which CBD oil can help with some symptoms.

Alzheimer's disease is a progressive mental deterioration that can occur in middle or old age, due to generalized degeneration of the brain. It is the most common cause of premature senility.

Multiple sclerosis is a chronic and progressive disease. It involves damage to the nerve cells in a person's brain and spinal cord, which can include numbness, speech impairment, loss of muscular coordination, blurred vision, and severe fatigue.

Parkinson's disease affects the way you move. It happens when there is a problem with certain nerve cells in the brain.

STROKES

A stroke is the brain equivalent of a heart attack. It can happen to anyone at any time. It happens when blood flow to a part of your brain is cut off. When this happens, brain cells are deprived of oxygen and begin to die. When brain cells die during a stroke, abilities controlled by that area of the brain, such as memory and muscle control, are lost.

ANTI-ACNE

The effects of CBD on immune system receptors may help reduce overall inflammation in the body. In turn, CBD oil may offer benefits for acne management.

Some studies have investigated the role of CBD in preventing cancer cell growth, but research is still in its early stages. The National Cancer Institute (NCI) says that CBD may help alleviate cancer symptoms and cancer treatment side effects. However, the NCI doesn't fully endorse any form of cannabis as a cancer treatment.

Patients with cancer or neurological diseases often benefit from a balanced ratio of CBD and THC. Research has shown that a CBD-THC 1:1 ratio is most effective for neuropathic pain. Finding the right therapeutic use of cannabis requires a careful, step-by-step process of starting with small doses, observing the results and then gradually increasing the amount of THC.

For cancer patients to increase appetite, try 2.5 mg of THC with or without 1 mg of CBD for six weeks.

Anti-inflammatory (Healing Inflammation)

A number of studies on CBD indicate that it may be useful for treating inflammation associated with a variety of conditions.

Anecdotal reports and early studies suggested that CBD may be of value in treating epilepsy, but the quality of the studies was too poor to draw definitive conclusions. But I am sure you all have seen the show on CNN where Dr. Sanjay Gupta showed a little girl with epilepsy and her family, and how they were able to find healing from Cannabis derived medicine. In case you haven't seen it, here is a link to that video.

https://www.youtube.com/watch?v=vyf-ffoatHg

Dosage: 200-300mg of CBD for up to 4 1/2 months.

WEIGHT-RELATED ILLNESSES

Weight-related illnesses can occur when you weigh more than your body can actually handle, and the end result can be many adverse consequences, such as heart disease, diabetes, body inflammation and soreness, and many others. CBD oil can help you lose weight, which could help rectify these serious symptoms in your body.

CBD was found to stimulate the expression of genes and proteins that enhance the breakdown and oxidation of fat.

This means that as you eat, your body stores less of the fat you consume. It can increase your body's ability to burn calories. You can burn more calories doing the same activities you would do in your daily life. Finally, CBD oil can also decrease the expression of proteins involved in fat cell generation.

The idea of losing weight with the help of cannabis is becoming very popular, and already there's talk of "cannabis diets." CBD might really boost metabolism, helping people to lose weight

CHRONIC PAIN MANAGEMENT

Chronic and severe pain presents a serious public health issue all around the world. Chronic pain is pain that lasts for more than 3 months. In the U.S., about 20% of adults suffer from chronic pain. Doctors are always looking for new medical options to help reduce chronic pain in sufferers. However, they will always be under constant scrutiny for their prescription practices. The introduction of CBD-related medication into the mainstream could provide hope to the millions of patients who suffer from chronic and acute pain.

Many researchers argue that CBD reacts positively with your immune system and receptors in your brain. This relationship can create anti-inflammatory and pain-relieving effects. Consequently, CBD oil can help with chronic pain management, such as for people with chronic back pain.

It is worth noting that CBD oil has also helped people with chronic menstrual cramps. However, the dosage varies from person to person. Patients with chronic migraines also cited immediate relief with few side effects after using CBD oil as compared to pharmaceutical drugs.

Dosage: For chronic pain - 2.5-20 mg CBD for an average of 25 days.

DOSAGE FOR OTHER ILLNESSES

For movement problems such as Huntington's disease, 10 mg of CBD per kg (2 lbs.) of weight for six weeks.

For sleep disorders - 40-160 mg CBD.

For multiple sclerosis - 2.5-120mg of a THC-CBD combination for 2-15 weeks.

For schizophrenia - 40-1,280mg CBD for up to four weeks.

For glaucoma, a single dose of 20-40mg of CBD.

BIPHASIC EFFECT

All cannabis compounds have a biphasic property. This means that a low and high dose of the same substance will have opposite effects. Small doses of cannabis often stimulate, while large doses sedate. While not lethal, too much THC can amplify anxiety and mood disorders.

CBD doesn't have any known adverse side effects at any dose, but drug interactions can present an issue. Too much CBD could be less effective than a moderate dose.

Always remember when it comes to cannabis therapy, less is more, is often the best approach.

POTENTIAL SIDE EFFECTS OF CBD OIL

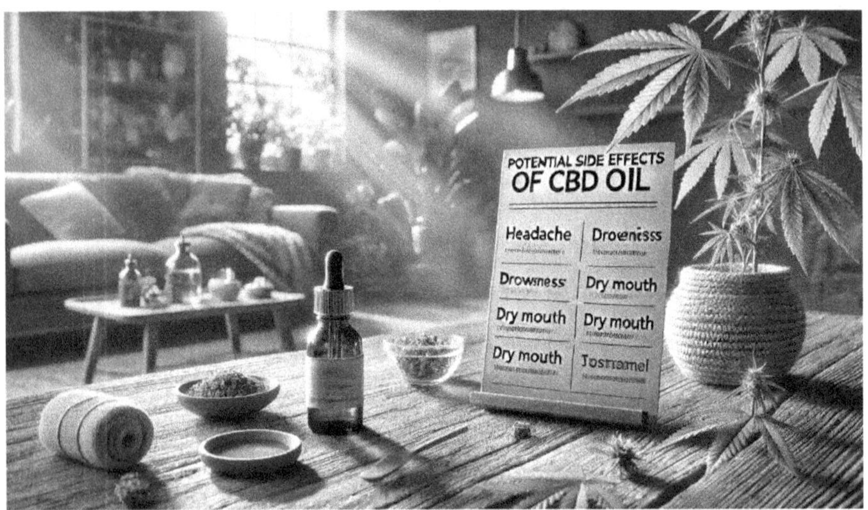

Just like anything you consume, especially medicines, there are side effects. Some are worse than others, and everyone responds differently. It is important to consider these side effects before starting CBD oil and to watch for them after you begin taking it regularly.

Inhibition of hepatic drug metabolism and decreased activity of p-glycoprotein are the first side effects we will discuss today. This means that CBD oil can really affect how your body absorbs your other medicines. It can slow your body's absorption or prevent it altogether. This can be tough for individuals who seek to begin a CBD regimen but are fearful of this side effect.

Consult with your doctor. They may be able to work with you in order to find a method that allows you to use CBD oil and avoid this side effect. This is a side effect that is prevalent in hemp oil as well. It is also what consuming grapefruit can do to your body. Because of this, you and your doctor should be able to work out a safe plan.

Dry mouth is a very commonly reported symptom of using CBD oil is dry mouth. This is more of an uncomfortable than a serious symptom. Dry mouth is an unpleasant sensation of dryness in the mouth. This effect appears to result from the endocannabinoid system's role in inhibiting saliva secretion. Dry mouth will pretty much just make you thirsty. If you have this symptom for too long, it could allow more bacteria to grow in your mouth, which can negatively affect you.

To mitigate this symptom, you can purchase a mouth rinse specifically designed for those with dry mouth.

These rinses have been proven to be very helpful. There are other oral products that can help you as well. Take some time to research and find the best method for you. If it is particularly inconvenient, talk to your doctor to see what other options are available for you.

CBD oil may or may not be effective for those suffering from Parkinson's disease. In some studies, the results have shown that CBD taken in high doses may worsen tremor and muscle movement in Parkinson's disease sufferers. However, there are also studies that suggest that CBD oil is safe and tolerated very well by patients affected by this condition. If you are thinking about treating someone with Parkinson's disease with CBD oil, contact their doctor and seek their advice. If, after using CBD oil, negative side effects or worsening symptoms are observed, the dose should be reduced or eliminated altogether to mitigate these potential side effects.

Higher doses of CBD oil can cause a small drop in blood pressure, usually within a few minutes of the CBD entering your system. This drop in blood pressure is often associated with lightheadedness. This can be especially dangerous if you are operating a motor vehicle or at work.

If you are already taking medication for blood pressure, don't start a CBD oil regimen before talking to your doctor to see if it will be safe for you to do so. This side effect of CBD is temporary and can often be resolved by drinking a cup of coffee or tea. It is essential to look out for signs of lightheadedness so you can take appropriate action.

Similar to lightheadedness, higher doses of CBD can cause drowsiness. If you are affected this way, you should not operate machinery or drive a vehicle. If you are experiencing drowsiness, you might have difficulty keeping your eyes open.

You might also slur your words or have trouble following a conversation. If you are experiencing regular drowsiness, contact your doctor. You and your doctor can work together to determine whether it is, in fact, the CBD oil causing your drowsiness or if there is another reason. It is also important to note that, in most cases, however, CBD is a wake-inducing agent.

Some common side effects are:

- ➤ Tiredness
- ➤ Diarrhea
- ➤ Appetite changes
- ➤ Weight gain or loss

When you use CBD oil with other medications, it can make them more or less effective. If you are going to think about using CBD oil, then you should discuss its use with your doctor. Doctors may want to monitor you for any changes while you take CBD oil and adjust your other medications as needed.

It is also important to note that the long-term effects of CBD oil have yet to be studied. Perhaps one of the biggest areas that hasn't been researched enough is CBD's effect on hormones.

FREQUENTLY ASKED QUESTIONS

What is CBD Oil Produced From?

CBD oil is extracted from the leaves, stalks, and flowers of the hemp plant.

Is It Legal?

Since CBD oil doesn't contain the psychoactive properties of THC, it is legal.

Do You Need a Prescription?

While you don't need a prescription for CBD oil, you should discuss taking it with your doctor to make sure it is okay to take with your other medications or health conditions.

How Long Does It Take to Take Effect?

This will depend on the extract and dosage. At the right dose, it can take between 20 and 30 minutes to see noticeable effects. It will also be affected by your specific health condition.

PART -2
HEMP OIL

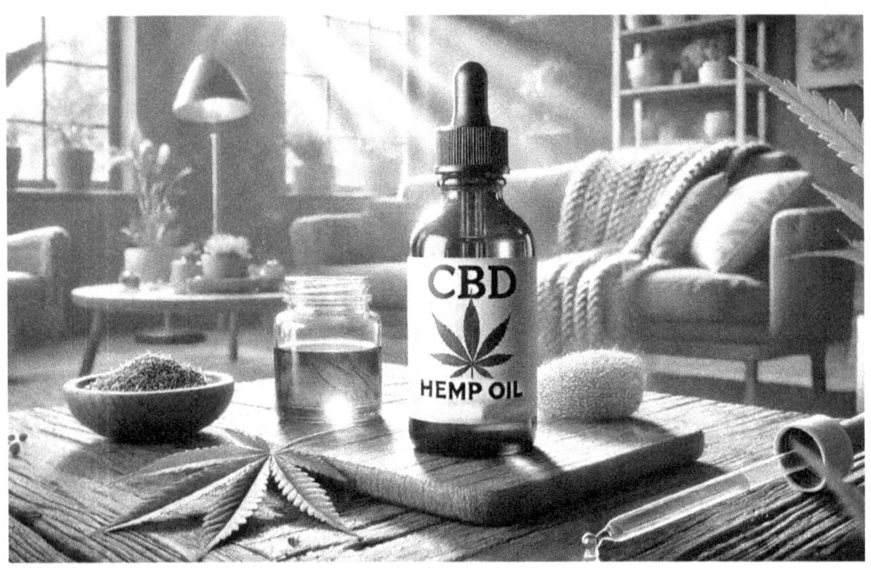

As I discussed earlier, hemp and CBD are different, even though they are often lumped together. This section is all about the best hemp strains and what makes them great.

1. CHARLOTTE'S WEB

This strain is an amazing one for hemp. It is completely organic. It has a CBD/THC ratio of 20:1. This strain became popular with its namesake, a 5-year-old girl named Charlotte, who used this strain to overcome the more than 50 seizures a day that she suffered through. The high CBD content of this plant makes it ideal for hemp use.

2. JAMAICAN LION

This strain is amazing for hemp extraction. But only in specific time frames. Harvesting after the 9th week will yield a product with a CBD/THC ratio of 13:1; before that, the ratio is 1:1. It is a hybrid of Mountain Lion and Yardies. It is great for cognitive health and relief from stress or anxiety.

3. AVI-DEKEL

This strain has a 16:1 CBD/THC ratio. It is as close to zero as it could be. It's one of the most well-known and consistently good hemp strains. It is one of the very few strains that the FDA has given special permission for medical testing. It is a strain that works well for things such as nausea and stress. This strain is also commonly used in conjunction with cancer treatments.

4. STEPHEN HAWKING KUSH

This strain is great for daytime pain relief. It is often praised for its ability to help people relax and experience substantial pain relief. It can make users feel soothed, relaxed, and happy.

Cannabis Strain	Best Benefit	Fragrance
Charlotte's Web	Ideal for those with Chronic Pain and potential seizures	Flowery and sweet
Jamaican Lion	Stress-relieving strain	Tropical and nutty
Avi-dekel	Decreases stress and reduces nausea	Woody and piney

| Stephen Hawking Kush | Pain relieving, induces happy feelings | Tea, and woody |

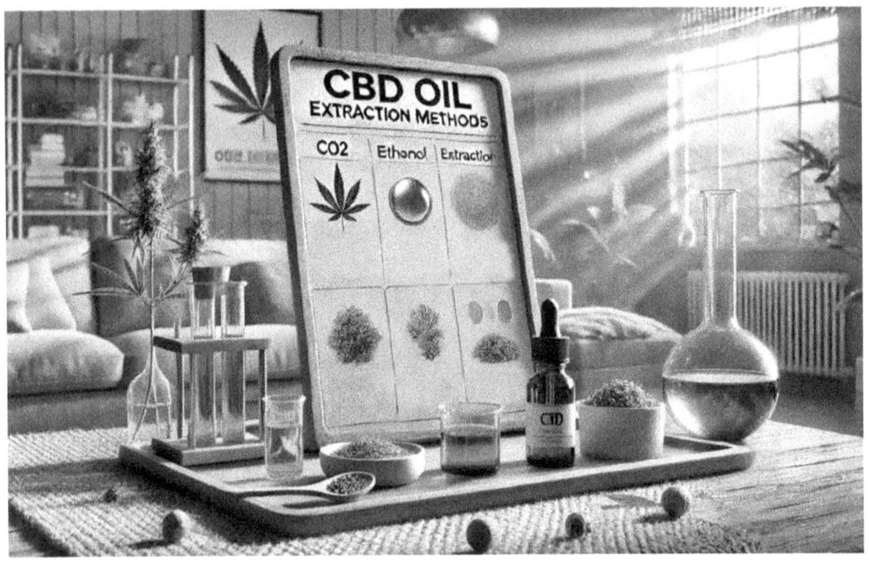

There are several extraction methods, and they don't require much equipment. It's important to remember that some of these methods might be simple, but they are not safe. It involves flammable liquids and fumes. It should therefore only be undertaken with great care and consideration. This process creates what is commonly known as Rick Simpson Oil. It should be created only by those with a medical marijuana license

Here's what you need to get started:

- 1 ounce of marijuana that is high in CBD, 2 plastic buckets
- 1 wooden stick
- 500 ML Isopropyl alcohols
- 1 coffee filter
- 1 large container
- 1 rice cooker
- 1 ventilation fan
- 1 tsp water
- Oven mitts or tea towels
- 1 stainless steel bowl
- A coffee warmer
- 1 glass bottle

Here's what you'll need to do:

1. Make sure your marijuana is completely dry. Place it in a plastic bucket.

2. Dampen the marijuana with 99% isopropyl alcohol.

3. Crush the dampened hemp with the wooden stick.

4. Add more alcohol until the material is just covered, then mix for three minutes. This will get about 80% of the CBD to dissolve off the plant into the alcohol.

5.   You need to do the second round to get the remaining 20%. Pour the oil and alcohol mix into the other bucket. Then add more alcohol to just about cover the plant material and mix for three minutes.

6.   Add this alcohol mix to another bucket and dispose of the plant material.

7.   Pour your mix through a coffee filter into a new container.

8.   It's now time to boil the alcohol off. This is the time to use the rice cooker.

The fumes from this process are highly flammable and toxic. Do not breathe them in. You do NOT want to breathe them in. Set up in a well-ventilated space with a good fan to help blow the fumes away. Make sure you keep away from any sparks, cigarettes, naked flames, hot elements, or anything that could ignite the fumes.

9. Fill the rice cooker to around the 3/4 mark. Turn it to high heat, keeping the temperature no higher than 290°F.

10.   As the alcohol dissolves, level of the mixture will drop in the rice cooker. Once it is lower than the ¾ mark,

keep adding the rest of your alcoholic mixture until it's all in.

11. When there is only about 1 inch left in the rice cooker, add a teaspoon of water to the mixture. This helps release any leftover alcohol residue and protect the oil from overheating.

12. Using your oven mitts, pick up your rice cooker. Then gently stir the mixture until the solvent has completely evaporated.

13. You can now pour your oil into a clean container.

14. Now, place your container on a gentle heating device like a coffee warmer for several hours. This is an important step because it allows the remaining water and alcohol to evaporate from the oil.

15. Watch the oil, and after it has stopped bubbling, it's ready! Just pour it into a clean bottle, and you're good to go.

Keep in mind that some strains can produce very thick oil, which can be difficult to squeeze out. If this happens, simply place a kitchen syringe in hot water for a couple of minutes, then use it to fill the clean bottle.

While extracting your own CBD or Hemp oil does work well, you might find the simplest method is to purchase these products.

There are many reputable online and physical retailers to choose from. Make sure you do your due diligence; not every retailer has your best interests at heart, nor is everyone honest about the products they sell. Choose licensed dealers every time.

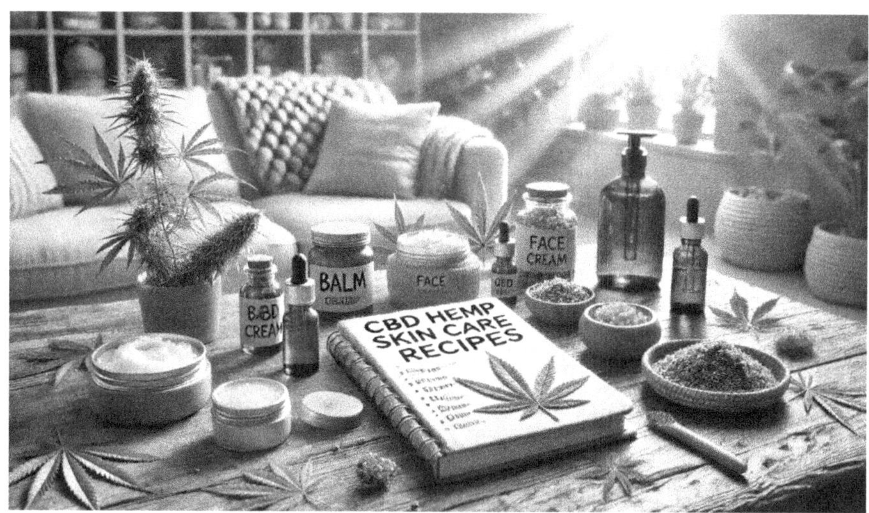

NATURAL HEMP OIL SHAMPOO RECIPE

Hemp oil is a wonderful natural moisturizer. It can also enhance hair growth due to the natural fatty acids it contains. This is a simple recipe that makes about a liter of natural hemp shampoo.

Here's what you will need:

3 1/2 cups of water

1 cup of castile soap

1 1/4 tsp of hemp oil

The process to create this shampoo is very simple. It only uses a few ingredients and takes about ten minutes. After you are done, you will have enough shampoo to last a long while.

To make this shampoo, you take a large bowl that can easily fit all of the water and other ingredients. Pour the water in the bowl and add the castile soap. You'll want to mix this vigorously.

Finally, add the hemp oil, and mix completely.

HEMP OIL SUGAR SCRUB

This sugar scrub feels decadent and smells amazing. Using it will lead to smoother and better-smelling skin. It is also pretty easy to make and will last you a long time.

Here's what you'll need:

1 cup of loosely packed Organic Coconut Sugar

1/2 cup of Organic Coconut Oil (in solid form)

1/3 cup of Organic Hemp Oil

1 ½ tablespoons of unsweetened organic cocoa powder

10 drops of essential oil of your choice:

To make this sugar scrub, simply combine all the ingredients in a large bowl and mix until well combined.

If you are having trouble combining it all, use the back of a spoon or a spatula to break down the coconut oil chunks.

To enjoy the scrub, simply rub it into your skin in small circular motions, then rinse off. This is not a face cleanser, so stick to your body only.

As you rub it into your skin, it will get a bit dry. When this happens, wet your hands and continue scrubbing for an even better polish.

THE ULTIMATE HEMP MASSAGE OIL

Massage oils sometimes come with ingredients that could irritate your skin. Making your own will allow you to customize your massage oil to your needs and enjoy the additional benefits of hemp oil.

<u>Here's what you'll need:</u>

10 drops of geranium oil

2 Tbsp. of jojoba oil

10- 20 drops of essential oils

The desired amount of CBD oil

This is an incredibly easy project. In a small container or plastic squeeze bottle, just combine all the oils with CBD oil. This oil can be used to massage sore muscles, as well as the hands and feet.

There isn't a part of your body that couldn't benefit from this mixture. Allow it to fully absorb into the skin before coming in contact with furniture or clothing.

HOMEMADE MOISTURIZING HEMP LIP BALM

Hemp oil is a great way to moisturize naturally. It works great in things like homemade moisturizing creams or lip balms. This is especially true if you have particularly dry skin or lips. Hemp oil prevents moisture loss while maintaining a proper moisture balance. It is also rich in vitamin D, which helps prevent skin aging and keeps it soft and hydrated.

<u>**Here's what you'll need:**</u>

1.5 teaspoon of beeswax

2 teaspoons of shea butter

2 teaspoons of hemp oil

3 drops of essential oil of your choice

<u>**Here's what you'll do:**</u>

1.   First, melt the beeswax and the shea butter in a double boiler.

2.   Turn off the heat to the double boiler and then add hemp oil along with your essential oils. Stir well. Make sure to do this while the mixture is still on the stove, so the mixture doesn't cool and harden. You will need to be quick to avoid any hardening.

3.   Now, pour the mixture into your lip balm containers. A great tool for this is a pipette, so you don't make a mess. If you don't have one, just pour it very carefully.

4.   Leave it to cool down for 15 minutes, and then you can use it.

The lip balm can last for at least a year.

ASK THESE QUESTIONS WHEN BUYING CBD OR HEMP OIL

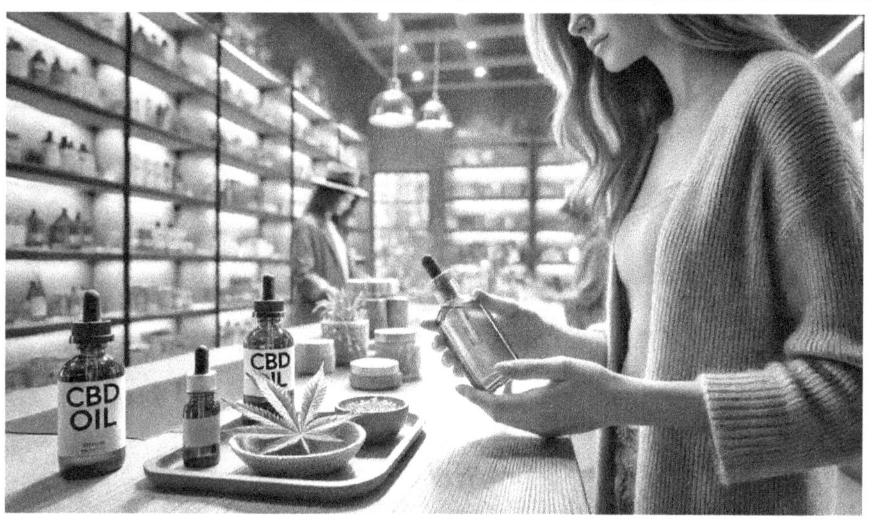

First, it is essential to ask about extraction methods.

Some retailers choose cheaper options that are considerably less safe than others. This is because many of those options are cheap. So if a retailer answers your question by saying they use propane or butane, that is not the retailer for you. Some retailers might tell you that these methods are their way of staying true to the plant's properties. However, this isn't true. Stay away from any retailer that uses these harsh products for extraction.

When purchasing CBD oil, look for Supercritical (or subcritical) CO2 extraction. This method uses carbon dioxide under high pressure and extremely low temperatures to isolate, preserve, and maintain the purity of the medicinal oil. While this method is more expensive and involves complex equipment and expertise, it ensures quality.

It's also eco-friendly and non-flammable, creating a safer laboratory and manufacturing environment, as well as better product control

When buying CBD oil or hemp oil, the source matters. The quality is really based on its source. By source, I mean where it was grown, how it was grown, and what the species of cannabis is. It also means the soil and climate. The main reason why hemp's cultivation environment is so important is that the cannabis plant easily absorbs contaminants from the soil while it grows.

So, the CBD oil you receive will have absorbed the environment in which the hemp was grown. This could yield a less-than-superior product because of it. So, ask questions to learn where the product you are buying comes from.

Bioavailability is also very important. CBD can be truly amazing. However, it is a very pricey solution for those who really need it. Maximizing bioavailability is essential to reducing costs for people. Bioavailability is basically how effective a single dose of CBD oil is, or how strong it is.

The stronger the CBD, the longer it will last. When buying CBD oil, ask about dosage and product strength, then try a few variations to find the best options for you. To increase the bioavailability of CBD oil, try eating some fat or oil, like a handful of nuts or full-fat yogurt, to improve absorption.

Cannabinoids are fat-loving molecules. They are readily taken up in the small intestine with a bit of dietary fat.

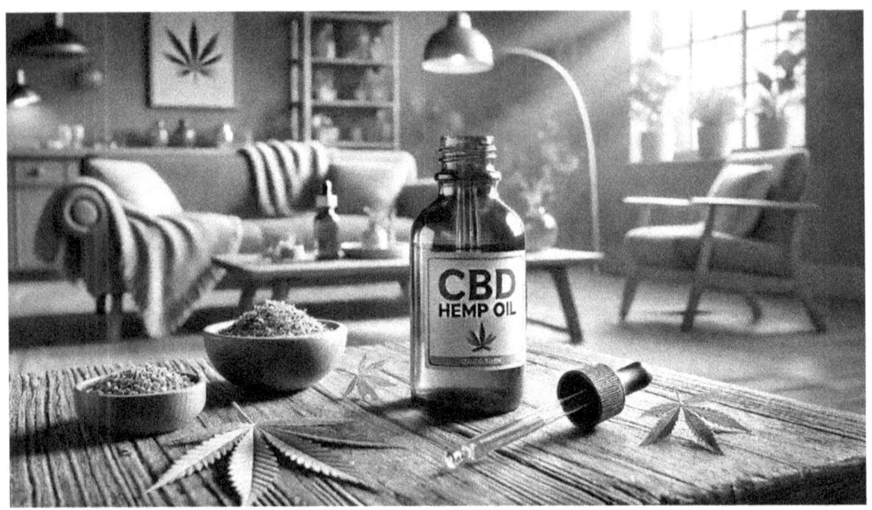

Hemp Oil Can Lower the Risk of Heart Disease

When it comes to hemp oil, researchers have discovered that specific organic compounds found in plants are responsible for lowering cholesterol in the oil. These compounds are responsible for this potential prevention of heart-related issues. Hemp oil can also reduce the risk of degenerative heart diseases and other conditions.

Use Hemp Oil to Reduce Inflammation

Hemp oil contains a variety of plant sterols and alcohols. These compounds have been shown to reduce inflammation.

Hemp Oil Relieves the Pain of Arthritis

Also related to the reduction of inflammation, consumption of hemp oil has been associated with relief from arthritis pain.

It Helps Prevent Some Forms of Cancer

Due to its omega-3 fatty acid profile, hemp oil naturally balances inflammation levels and helps strengthen your immune system. Hemp oil offers some cancer prevention properties, too.

Use Hemp Oil to Heal Skin Conditions

Hemp oil has also been found to help heal skin conditions such as eczema, psoriasis and other rashes. The oil's fatty acids are believed to affect immune responses in the body, helping promote healing. This is also likely due to the oil's perfect balance of omega-6 and omega-3 fatty acids.

Hemp Oil for a Healthy Complexion

Hemp oil is great for giving your skin a beautiful complexion. It is very easily absorbed and moisturizing without being greasy. The oil can help to clean and detoxify skin, as well as even out skin tone.

Unlike many other oils, hemp oil can nourish dry skin without making it overly oily. It won't clog pores as easily as other heavier oils. So, if you're looking for a good moisturizer, consider hemp oil. Hemp oil is similar to our skin's natural lipids. Thus, it can penetrate cells to deeply moisturize both the epidermis and subdermal layers.

Hemp Oil Treats Acne

You might not think that using any oil would be good for treating acne. However, because of its light consistency, hemp oil is perfect for acne-prone skin as it's not greasy at all. One great way to use hemp oil is to mix it with other skin-healing oils. You can also add a couple of drops of lavender oil or other essential oils. This mixture can help clear your skin without clogging your pores.

Hemp Oil Supports Weight Loss

Substituting hemp oil for other oils in your diet can even help you lose weight. It reduces sugar cravings, helping lower your calorie intake and curb inflammation. You can try adding hemp oil to a breakfast smoothie to help curb excessive hunger throughout the day.

It's a Great Source of Plant-Based Protein

Vegans and vegetarians can sometimes have a hard time getting enough protein in their diets without meat. Adding hemp oil is a great way to accomplish this, as it provides a similar amount of protein to that found in meat. About 25% of the calories from the oil come from protein.

Use Hemp Oil for Beautiful Hair

Hemp oil offers benefits to the hair as well. It can help your hair grow beautifully and increase shine. There are many recipes for homemade conditioners, shampoos, and other hair products that call for the oil. Using hemp oil on the scalp can help improve blood circulation and prevent scalp infections.

Using these products can result in stronger, healthier and longer hair growth. It can also help thicken hair texture. Hemp oil can prevent dandruff and reduce hair loss. When applied directly to the ends, it can moisturize and strengthen strands, helping prevent breakage.

SIDE EFFECTS OF HEMP

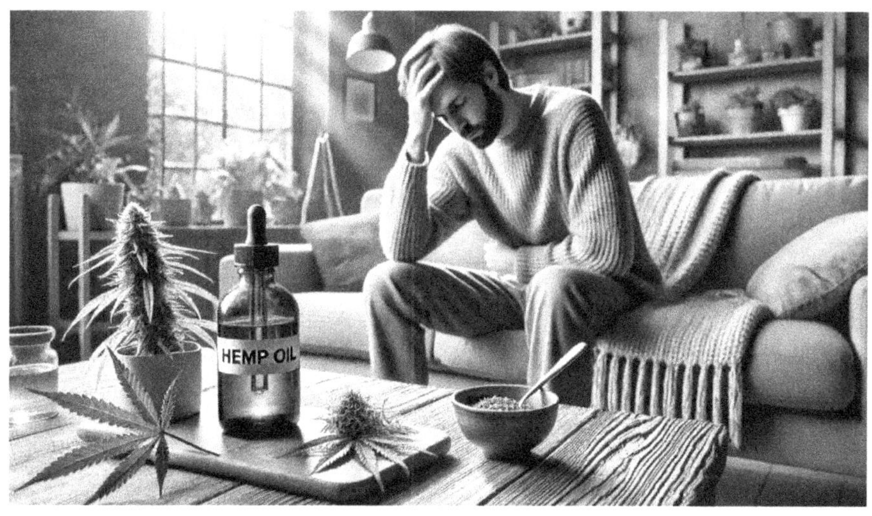

Hemp oil, as the name suggests, is processed from the seeds as well as the actual hemp plant. It has nearly none of the psychoactive THC element, which is the primary difference between CBD and THC. In fact, hemp oil is rich in omega fatty acids, which are found in foods like fish and olive oil.

However, hemp oil isn't entirely free of side effects, and it's important to be aware of the possibilities. While most people never experience any significant, unexpected effects, knowing them beforehand will help you deal with anything that may come up.

HEMP OIL CONTAINS POLYUNSATURATED FATTY ACIDS

The omega-3's in hemp oil are very beneficial to the body. However, there can be consequences when they are taken in excess. If your body has an excess of fatty acids, then you are susceptible to several issues, including cardiac dysfunction and increased susceptibility to bacterial infections.

When exposed to intense heat, hemp oil produces harmful peroxides

Heating hemp oil above 121 degrees F breaks down the fatty acids into harmful peroxides. If you are exposed to this compound, you could get hurt. It can damage your skin and other organs, as well as the areas around you. If hemp oil is heated above the threshold, then there is the probability of the compound exploding and causing fires.

So hemp oil should only be used on warm and cold dishes, unless combined with other substances that mitigate this risk, such as the ingredients in baked goods. Remember, hemp oil is natural, so it's perishable just like other natural products. Keeping your oil in an airtight container, preferably in the fridge, is the best way to ensure its longevity.

HEMP OIL USE CAN LEAD TO DIGESTIVE PROBLEMS FOR SOME PEOPLE

Some people experience stomach problems when using hemp oil. Some of these symptoms include soft stools, diarrhea, and painful cramps. If you are susceptible to stomach issues, make sure that you consult your doctor before taking hemp oil.

HEMP OIL IS STILL PSYCHOACTIVE IN OVERLY SENSITIVE INDIVIDUALS

Even though the amount of the psychoactive element of THC in hemp oil is ordinarily pretty negligible, there are some people who still get a high sensation after consuming it. This may lead to serious issues such as hallucinations and anxiety. If you are overly sensitive to THC, stop using hemp oil immediately and don't consume any more without seeking the opinion of your doctor.

Keep in mind that there are many different hemp oil products, and they contain different levels of THC. It could be a good idea to try different forms of CBD to find one that works for you. However, the amount of THC is generally low enough that many people won't notice any psychoactive effects at all.

HEMP OIL MAY LEAD TO BLOOD CLOTTING

Hemp oil can affect how anticoagulants and blood platelets work in your body. It can sometimes even stop their production. Blood platelets are essential in the blood clotting process. Because of this possibility, if you have an issue with blood clotting, you should not consume hemp oil until after you consult with your doctor.

MITIGATING CBD SIDE EFFECTS

To put it simply, the best way to mitigate the side effects of hemp oil is to lower your dose—the lower the levels of hemp oil in your body, the lower the chance you'll experience side effects. However, since the side effect profile is so small, consider gradually increasing your dose until you find the right balance for you.

While most people experience little to no side effects from hemp, it's important to know the risks involved before you start using hemp oil. Without this information, people may not realize that CBD oil is the actual cause. They might think that a symptom is being caused by hemp oil when it's actually something else.

Pay attention, and if you notice any unexpected effects, talk to your doctor about your next steps and ways to reduce them. We, as people, respond in unique ways based on many factors. After you've had a chance to try a few things out, you'll be able to find something that gives you all the benefits you need with the fewest drawbacks possible.

CBD AND FEDERAL LAW

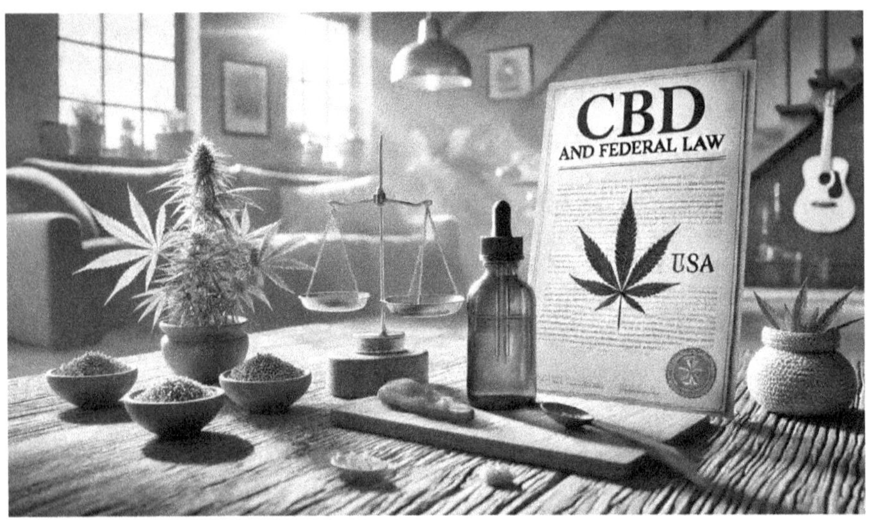

Within the cannabis universe, there are two types of plants that are very broadly categorized: hemp and drug plants. Hemp plants include any plant grown for fiber or seed oil. Drug plants include THC-rich psychoactive plants and non-psychoactive CBD-rich plants. The difference in these two plants is the resin content. Most hemp plants are low in resin, while drug plants are typically high in resin.

Industrial hemp is often a low-resin agricultural crop grown from pedigree seeds. They are usually grown in clusters of 100 tall, skinny plants per square meter, then harvested by machine and manufactured into products such as textiles and paper.

Drug plants are a high-resin crop that is often grown from asexually reproduced clones at one to two plants per square meter. These plants are hand-harvested, dried, trimmed and cured.

RESIN LAWS

At one time, federal law defined marijuana based on its resin content. In the 1970 Controlled Substances Act, the resin was mentioned three times within the definition of marijuana.

The law stated that while certain parts of the plant, such as the mature stalk and sterilized seed, are exempt from the legal definition of marijuana, flowers, leaves, and stick resin, wherever found on the plant, are not exempt.

Federal law is clear on the point that the resin from any part of the marijuana plant or any preparation made from the resin is not allowed under the law. The fiber produced from hemp stalks and the oil pressed from hemp seed are legal, but the resin isn't. A little confusing? Well, read on.

When it comes to the medicinal and recreational use of cannabis, the resin is the most commonly used portion. The resin contains both THC and CBD, along with some other components, as I discussed at the start of this book.

The resin is found within the heads of tiny, mushroom-shaped trichomes on the female flowers or buds. To a lesser extent, some resin can be found on the leaves.

THE THC ISSUE

It is clear that since the beginning, the Federal government assumed resin content was the main factor in separating marijuana from industrial hemp. However, federal law has changed to include a caveat that officially characterizes industrial hemp as nothing containing more than 0.3% THC by dry weight. This small amount of THC won't have any euphoric effect.

This figure comes from a 1976 taxonomic report by Canadian scientists Ernest Small and Arthur Cronquist. The 0.3% figure was never intended to serve as a legal definition, but it eventually did. The Drug Enforcement Administration started everything by trying to ban hemp food products, including hemp seed oil.

On October 9, 2001, the DEA published an "Interpretative Rule." This states that any product containing any amount of THC is classified as a Schedule 1 controlled substance. This effort fell apart due to the actions of the Hemp Industries Association (HIA). In February 2004, the HIA won when the Ninth Circuit Court of Appeals rejected the ban on hemp food based on substantive grounds.

However, this court decision didn't affect the legal status of CBD. The Controlled Substances Act remained the law.

Although CBD hemp oil purveyors often cited the February 2004 ruling as a basis for claiming that their products are legal in all states. The court decision never mentioned CBD, and many maintain that the ruling didn't legalize CBD.

THE FARM BILL

The 2004 court decision also didn't mention anything about a THC percentage. It wasn't until ten years later that the Federal Farm Bill was passed. Also known as the Agricultural Act of 2014, this law added the 0.3% THC rule to federal law.

Section 7606 of the Agricultural Act included the definition for industrial hemp for the first time in US history and provided a clear distinction between marijuana. Cannabis was classified as hemp, not marijuana, as long as no part of the plant exceeded the 0.3% concentration of THC.

Section 7606 of the Farm Bill didn't mention resin, thereby creating a legal exception for growing industrial hemp in the United States under state-approved pilot research programs. This loophole opened opportunities for industrial hemp advocates.

For the first time in many years, American farmers could cultivate industrial hemp on domestic soil on a provisional basis, rather than relying on hemp-grown products from abroad for marketing in the United States. However, it was limited to states that legalized industrial hemp farming. Growing industrial hemp outside of state-sanctioned pilot research is still not allowed by federal law.

(Information found in this section is taken from the Project CBD website: https://www.projectcbd.org/about/cannabis-facts/sourcing-cbd-marijuana-industrial-hemp-vagaries-federal-law)

There are many hemp products called "Hemp Extract oil" and "Hemp Oil." Is there a difference?

No, these are just different terms that are used by brands in the CBD industry. If you're confused about whether the product you want to buy is CBD oil, make sure to confirm with your chosen retailer so you know exactly what you are getting. However, do not confuse CBD oil with hemp oil, which is different.

What is the difference between CBD Oil and Hemp Oil?

Hemp Oil is derived from hemp seeds and is primarily used for dietary purposes. Refined hemp oil can also be used in beauty care products, as they have amazing skin care properties. CBD oil is not the same thing as hemp oil. It is extracted from one of hemp's cannabinoids. They have different properties.

Can I give CBD oil to my dog or cat?

There are retailers that sell pet-safe CBD oil brands. They have been known to help animals with anxiety. Make sure you do your research and consult with a vet before giving your pet CBD oil.

Do I need a doctor's prescription or a medical marijuana card (Red Card)?

No, since hemp-derived CBD products are dietary supplements. There is no need to obtain a doctor's recommendation or to live in a medical marijuana state to have these products delivered to your door.

What's the difference between marijuana CBD oil and industrial hemp CBD oil?

The main difference between marijuana CBD and hemp CBD is the differences in levels of THC the oil contains. Marijuana CBD oil typically contains a high level of THC along with CBD, which means that it is psychoactive. Hemp CBD, on the other hand, has a high level of CBD with a minimal amount of THC

Don't you need some THC to synergize with CBD?

There is no reliable scientific evidence that THC is necessary to synergize the effects of CBD. The best CBD oil is the one with as little THC as possible.

What is the best way to produce CBD-rich cannabis oil?

To extract CBD-rich cannabis oil, you have to start with a plant that is CBD-rich. As you read in earlier chapters, there are many ways to extract oil from the cannabis plant. Each extraction method has its pros and cons. Some methods are safer and more effective than others. Many methods require expensive equipment and extensive expertise, but two are safe for a realistic home extraction. These two are oil extractions and dry ice extraction.

Using another method at home can result in dangerous consequences, such as explosions, skin damage, or fires. It is best to stick to the safe methods described in this book so you can achieve the results you want without taking any risks.

Can I get CBD from juicing raw cannabis?

Juicing or otherwise ingesting raw, unheated cannabis, will not get you the results you want or need. A CBD-rich strain contains CBD acid, which, when heated, becomes CBD. Without that heat, you will miss out on many of the benefits of CBD oil.

Is a CBD-dominant cannabis strain with very little THC a better medicine than a cannabis strain with a fifty-fifty CBD-THC mix?

The answer to this depends on why you are taking CBD oil. For many uses, the THC content doesn't make the CBD oil less useful. However, for specific ailments, use the cannabinoid strain that is the richest in CBD. This will have a very positive effect on the user. Two examples of this would be those that are seeking to treat anxiety and seizure disorders. However, those patients with pain syndromes and neurodegenerative disorders may benefit from a substantial amount of THC. It is up to the individual, based on their unique needs, to determine the right type of CBD oil for them.

Will I fail a drug test if I medicate with CBD Oil?

Yes, there is a significant chance that you will fail a drug test even if you experience no mood-altering effects from your CBD-rich medicine. Drug tests are geared toward identifying THC, not CBD or another cannabinoid. So, if you are going to take a drug test, it is best not to take CBD oil. Tests are geared to pick up on it.

Which is better, CBD extracted from cannabis or industrial hemp?

CBD-rich products are made using only organic cannabis hemp. The reason for this is that it offers the best safety and better medicinal benefits. The CBD products derived from industrial hemp can have several potential problems. The first being that it typically contains much less cannabidiol than CBD-rich cannabis strains. This means that it takes a much larger amount of industrial hemp to extract the same amount of CBD as organically grown hemp. Also, industrial hemp lacks the critical medicinal terpenes and secondary cannabinoids found in cannabis oil

Can a grower increase CBD content by manipulating environmental factors?

This is not the case. A plant cannot be made to be CBD-rich. To do this, it needs to have the right genetic makeup already. The ratio of CBD is genetically predetermined.

Is growing CBD-rich cannabis any different from growing THC-dominant cannabis?

No, the process is largely the same. Just like growing high-THC strains, harvesting time matters. If you harvest earlier or later, you can affect the plant's cannabinoid levels.

Does CBD affect other medications?

CBD can inhibit the enzymes involved in metabolizing many drugs. It is similar to grapefruit in that way. This is why doctors advise patients not to eat grapefruit for a short period around the time they take medication. In some situations, it may be a good idea for your doctor to monitor your blood levels while taking CBD.

Because CBD is non-psychoactive, does that make it legal?

No, it doesn't make it legal. In the United States, it is lumped in with marijuana and is completely illegal. This is despite its lack of addictive potential and strong safety profile. However, there are several states that have decriminalized and legalized Cannabidiol and all other plant cannabinoids. These laws are very fluid at the state level, so check your state's laws to better understand their status as where you live.

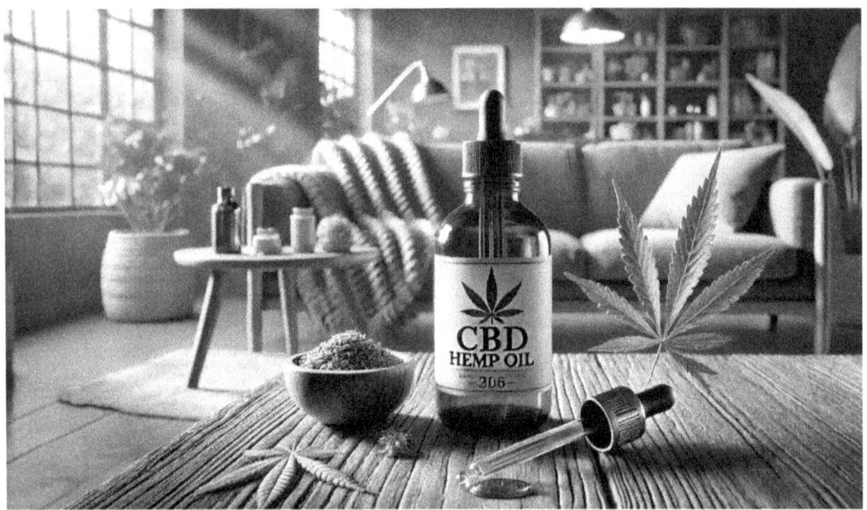

I want to THANK YOU for purchasing and reading this book. I really hope you got a lot out of it!

I LOVE getting feedback from my wonderful readers, and reviews really do make a difference. I read all of my reviews and would love to hear your thoughts.

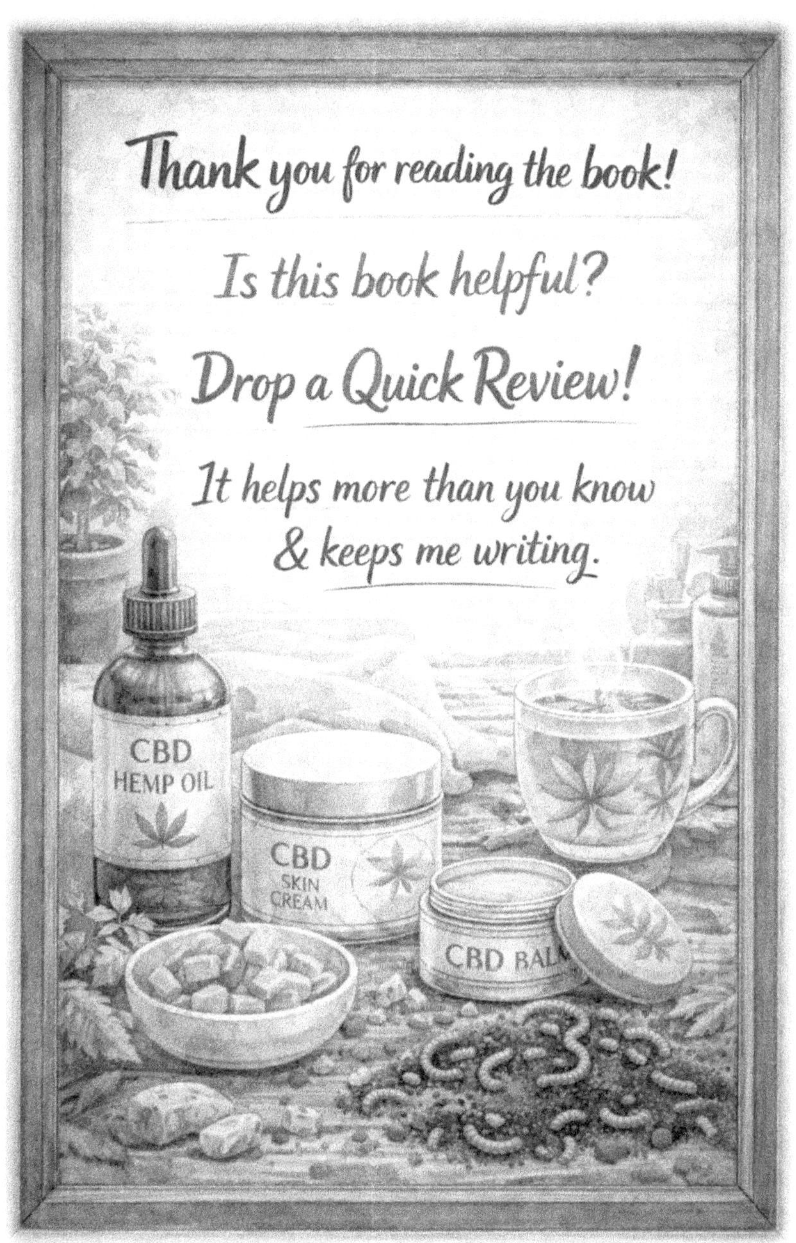

Thank you for reading the book!

Is this book helpful?

Drop a Quick Review!

It helps more than you know
& keeps me writing.

CBD
HEMP OIL

CBD
SKIN
CREAM

CBD BALM

www.ingramcontent.com/pod-product-compliance
Lightning Source LLC
Chambersburg PA
CBHW070123260726
48658CB00001B/241